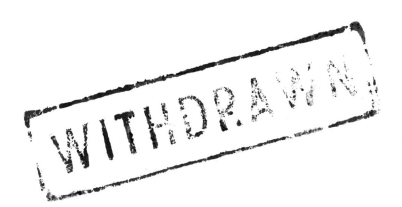

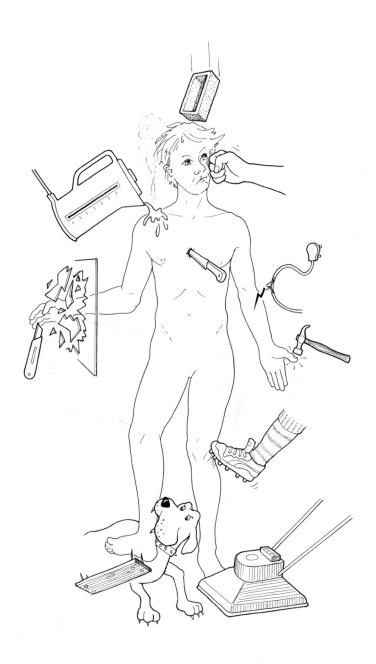

Modern 'wounded man'

OXFORD HANDBOOKS IN EMERGENCY MEDICINE
Series Editors R. N. Illingworth, C. E. Robertson, and M. J. Clancy

OXFORD HANDBOOKS IN EMERGENCY MEDICINE

This series covers topics of interest to all Accident and Emergency staff. The books are aimed at junior doctors and casualty nurses. Each book starts with an introduction to the topic, including epidemiology where appropriate. The clinical presentation and the immediate practical management of common conditions is described in detail, so that the casualty officer or nurse is able to deal with the problem on the spot. A specific course of action is recommended for each situation, and alternatives discussed.

The Management of Wounds and Burns

Second Edition

Jim Wardrope
Consultant, Accident and Emergency Medicine
Northern General Hospital, Sheffield

and

June A. Edhouse
Senior Registrar, Accident and Emergency Medicine
Northern General Hospital, Sheffield

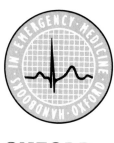

OXFORD
UNIVERSITY PRESS

OXFORD
UNIVERSITY PRESS

Oxford University Press, Great Clarendon Street, Oxford OX2 6DP
Oxford New York
Athens Auckland Bangkok Bogotá Buenos Aires Calcutta
Cape Town Chennai Dar es Salaam Delhi Florence Hong Kong Istanbul
Karachi Kuala Lumpur Madrid Melbourne Mexico City Mumbai
Nairobi Paris São Paulo Singapore Taipei Tokyo Toronto Warsaw
and associated companies in
Berlin Ibadan

Oxford is a trade mark of Oxford University Press

Published in the United States
by Oxford University Press, Inc., New York

© Jim Wardrope and June A. Edhouse, 1999

First edition, 1992

A catalogue record for this book is available from the British Library

Library of Congress Cataloging in Publication Data
(Data available)

ISBN 0 19 262999 9 (Pbk)

Typeset by Best-set Typesetter Ltd., Hong Kong
Printed in Great Britain by
Biddles Ltd., Guildford & King's Lynn

Preface

World-wide, millions of people each year still die from wounds and wound infections. The mortality in the United Kingdom from wounds is small. The high standard of Accident and Emergency care is one reason for this low mortality, along with excellent public health and high immunization rates.

Wound management is the 'bread and butter' of Accident and Emergency practice. In one year approximately three million wounds will be treated. Most of these wounds will appear minor and for many the treatment will be straightforward. However, proper wound assessment and management is essential, even in the most minor injuries. Disabling injury may be overlooked and life-threatening infections may follow inappropriate treatment.

Serious wounds that are an immediate threat to life are rare, but Accident and Emergency staff must be prepared to begin initial assessment and treatment until senior surgical help arrives.

Although most wound care is routine it should never be boring. Each wound is different and each individual will have different expectations regarding treatment. Remember the patient's point of view: 'the most important wound is the one that *I've* got'.

Sheffield   J. W.
1998   J. A. E.

Acknowledgements

We would like to thank all of those involved in the first edition of the book especially Mr J. A. R. Smith, and Mr Peter Cox for his work on the figures. We thank Mr G. Miller and Mr C. Caddy for their comments, Mr B. Tesfayohannes for advice on paediatric anaesthesia, and Mr N. Kidner for providing the additional illustrations for the figures.

We thank Mr G. Wilson and Convatec for permission to modify the burns chart (Fig. 11.2) and Professor B. Knight for permission to use Figure 1.3.

Contents

PART 1
Wound assessment

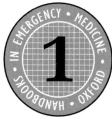

CHAPTER 1

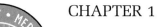

Wound assessment

Key points in wound assessment

1 History:
  (a) How?   Where?   When?
  (b) Tetanus, allergy, medical illness, medications.
2 Examination:
  (a) Wound size, type, depth, other features.
  (b) Integrity and function of other structures (especially nerves and tendons).
3 Investigations:
  (a) X-ray for fractures/foreign bodies/deep structure penetration.
  (b) Bacteriology—seldom indicated.
  (c) Blood—rarely: haematology/clotting.
4 Documentation:
  (a) Use diagrams ('one picture is worth a thousand words').
  (b) Record all findings (not written down = not done, in legal cases).

Introduction

Wounds may be life-threatening. Swift assessment and treatment are vital, and the initial management of such wounds is described in Chapter 2.

Some wounds will require immediate first aid, such as control of haemorrhage. This is achieved by direct pressure and elevation of the limb.

The vast majority of wounds presenting to the Accident and Emergency department will present no immediate threat to life. Therefore there SHOULD be plenty of time for thorough and accurate assessment of the wound, but the pressure of work may lead to 'corners being cut'. Although a wound may not be immediately life-threatening, mismanagement of wounds may lead to loss of life. There is no doubt that errors can lead to considerable permanent disability and costly litigation.

It is essential that full assessment is carried out. This need not be a lengthy process, but it is good practice to develop a routine, and this must include an accurate *history* and appropriate *examination*. Further *investigations* (most commonly X-rays) may be necessary for certain types of wound. All these findings must then be *recorded.*

Safe practice

Large numbers of wounds are seen every day in Accident and Emergency departments. Some patients will harbour blood-borne pathogens which pose a real threat to hospital staff.

- A&E staff should be immunized against hepatitis B
- Universal precautions must be applied
- Always wear gloves
- Wear mask/goggles if concerned about droplet spread
- Dispose of sharps safely. It is your responsibility to do so
- Clear up soiled dressing trays/suture packs after use
- Report any needlestick/inoculation injury to Occupational Health immediately

History

- How? Where? When?
- Tetanus/allergy/medical illness/medications
- Other factors • Non-accidental injury

A clear history is the cornerstone of accurate diagnosis. The first step in wound management is to try to visualize the exact *mechanism of injury* (**how**); the *environment* in which the injury occurred (**where**); and the *time* elapsed since wounding (**when**). The patient is asked about *tetanus* immunization status, *allergies*, and *medications* or *medical* conditions.

How?

You should persist in questioning the patient until the exact cause of the wound is clear. There are certain mechanisms of injury which give strong clues to diagnosis and treatment. See Figure 1.1.

Sharp implements and broken glass cut and penetrate tissue with great ease. If the wound was made by a sharp object then there should be an immediate suspicion that there will be injury to deeper structures. In vital areas such as the hand it is good practice to assume that deep structures have been damaged.

A history of a *crushing* type injury is very important, since the early examination may reveal little apart from tenderness. Such injuries cause much damage to the underlying tissues, sometimes resulting in fractures, but always resulting in tissue swelling, and often giving rise to troublesome long-term symptoms.

The suspicion that there might be a *foreign body* in the wound, such as metal, glass, or gravel, will indicate the need for radiography. It is best to ask the patient a direct question 'do you think there is any glass/metal/gravel in the wound?'

The history of a *bite* is very significant. The infection risk varies between species, but *human* bites carry great risk of

(a)   (b)

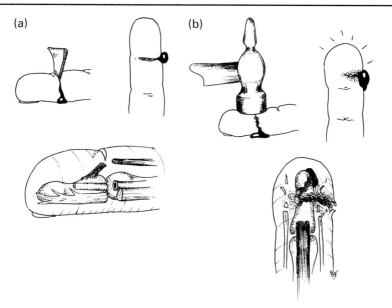

Fig. 1.1 . (a) The surface wound may appear small but there may be severe underlying damage. (b) Crushing may cause significant deformation at the time of injury. The apparently benign appearance does not reflect the degree of internal devastation to bone, soft tissue, and *especially* nerve.

bacterial infection, as well as the possibility of transmission of hepatitis B.

Any wound to the head or trunk carries the risk of life-threatening complications, and appropriate questioning should be used to elicit the associated symptoms of head, chest, or abdominal injury.

Where?

A wound sustained in the farmyard will have a high risk of contamination with the spores of *Clostridium tetani*. A wound sustained in the kitchen would not appear to have a high risk of tetanus contamination; yet a case of tetanus occurred in a young woman after cutting herself while peeling potatoes. The soil on the potato was the source of the infection. Elicit the *exact* environment in which the wound occurred.

It is fortunate that at present rabies is not endemic in the British Isles. It is vital that patients suffering animal bites abroad receive rabies prophylaxis (see p. 106).

When?

The greater the delay in obtaining proper wound care, the greater the chances of serious wound infection. If this interval is more than six hours then it should be assumed that bacteria have already begun to multiply and that the wound is infected. This should be considered when deciding on the best method of wound closure.

Tetanus, allergy, medical illness, medications

In busy accident and emergency departments it is inevitable that full detailed medical histories are not taken for every 'minor' injury. However, in the context of a patient with a wound there are four questions which are essential:

Tetanus immunization status
Allergies to drugs, dressings, local anaesthetics
Medical illness (e.g. valvular heart disease, joint prostheses, haemophilia, diabetes mellitus)
Medications: concurrent drug treatment, especially steroid or anticoagulant therapy

Some departments have prompt boxes incorporated into the A&E card to assist with the recording of this essential information (see Fig. 1.2).

Other factors

Consider other factors such as the patient's occupation and leisure interests, and if the wound involves the upper limb, whether the patient is left- or right-handed.

The functional demands of a labourer and a classical guitarist are very different and for certain hand wounds the best treatments for those individuals may be quite different. Similarly the cosmetic demands of a professional model and a front row rugby forward are likely to be different. In this

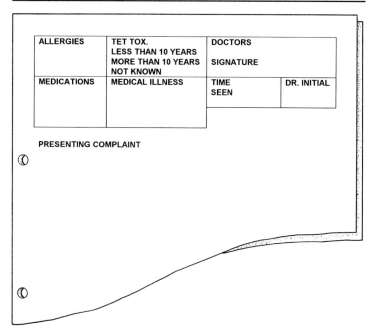

ALLERGIES	TET TOX. LESS THAN 10 YEARS MORE THAN 10 YEARS NOT KNOWN	DOCTORS SIGNATURE	
MEDICATIONS	MEDICAL ILLNESS	TIME SEEN	DR. INITIAL

PRESENTING COMPLAINT

Fig. 1.2 • Accident and Emergency card incorporating prompt boxes.

case the primary management may well be the same, but more intensive follow-up may be appropriate where cosmetic defects might be a problem.

Non-accidental injury

Children, females, and the elderly may present to the A&E department with an injury resulting from domestic abuse. They may not volunteer details of the incident. There is a duty to try to identity these patients, who may require more detailed investigation and follow-up.

It is the history and the interview with a patient or the carer that will lead to clues to the real cause of the injury.

> **Box 1.1 Indicators of possible non-accidental injury**
> 1. Delay between injury and seeking treatment.
> 2. The history of the accident does not fit with the observed injury.
> 3. The history changes.
> 4. Presence of other injuries, especially if at different stages of healing.
> 5. Signs of general neglect or failure to thrive.
> 6. Other indicators of family tension, the presence of financial problems or behavioural problems, an isolated single carer or single parent, or indications of alcohol or drug abuse.

If you feel that 'the story does not fit', then ask for more senior advice. Take more time over the history, and perform a full examination with the patient fully undressed.

More information on the family may be obtained from the general practitioner or social work department.

There is no single diagnostic factor for non-accidental injury. Such cases require an experienced, multidisciplinary approach to ensure the best outcome for the family.

Examination

- **Wound** • **Underlying structures**

The examination should consist of two distinct parts. The first is examination of the wound itself and the second is of the structures lying deep to the wound.

The wound. Wounds are painful and tend to bleed. It is essential to have the patient seated comfortably, and if there seems to be a risk of fainting then lie the patient down. Good light is essential.

1. *Measure* wounds accurately.
2. Areas of bruising or grazing and other features should be noted.

3. The depth may be difficult to assess. Wiping away blood clot will restart bleeding and cause pain. If you cannot assess the depth at this stage it *must* be done during the treatment of the wound.
4. Look for foreign bodies.

Underlying structures. No wound examination is complete without full examination of underlying structures which might be damaged. Further examination is performed to exclude such injury. For example, the examination of a head wound would not be complete without assessment of conscious level.

Think about *all* the structures which lie deep to the wound; vessels, nerves, tendons, bone, vital organs. Apply the appropriate clinical examination to detect any damage to these structures. More details of such examinations are given in the chapters dealing with wounds in specific areas.

Investigations

- **Radiography** • **Bacteriology** • **Blood investigations**

Most wounds will not require further investigation.
Radiography is the most common investigation.
Indications include:

- Crushing injury to exclude fracture
- Possibility of radiopaque foreign body (ask specifically for foreign body views)
- Possibility of joint penetration (e.g. wounds over knee)
- Significant trunk wound

If there is a possbility of a radiopaque foreign body in the wound then radiographs must be taken.

Table 1.1 indicates the materials likely to be radiopaque or radiolucent. *Ultrasound* can be useful in pinpointing radiolucent foreign bodies (e.g. wood).

Table 1.1 . Radiopaque/lucent materials

Radiopaque	Radiolucent
Glass	Wood
Metal	Most plastics
Gravel	
Teeth!	
Some plastics	
Ceramics/tiles	

Bacteriology

Wound swabs from fresh injuries are not needed. If a wound is infected then a swab may be indicated, although this seldom influences management. Wound swabs are advised if a wound is slow to heal, as low-grade infection can prevent epithelialization.

Blood investigations

If the blood loss has been large then a baseline haemoglobin concentration, haematocrit, and platelet count may be required. The results of these investigations will *not* give a reliable indication of the degree of blood loss.

If the patient is taking anticoagulant therapy or has a bleeding diathesis, and there is any difficulty achieving haemostasis, clotting studies should be performed.

Definitions and records
Definitions

Accurate descriptions of wounds require the correct usage of words, and appropriate definitions are given below (see also Fig. 1.3):

A wound *A breach in the external surface of the body*—in law the whole thickness of the skin should be breached.

Abrasion *A portion of surface from the skin that has been removed by rubbing (friction).*

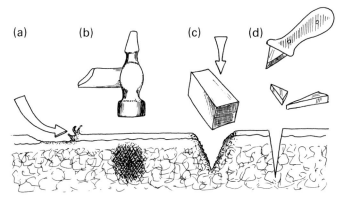

Fig. 1.3 • Terminology used to describe wounds. (a) Tangential force causing *abrasion*. (b) *Contusion*: no breach in the skin, underlying bruising. (c) *Laceration*: blunt violence causing tear in skin. (d) *Incised wound*: sharp implement causing breach in skin. (Adapted from *Forensic Pathology* by Professor B Knight, by kind permission of the author and Edward Arnold/Hodder & Stoughton Publishing.)

Cut (incised wound) *A breach in the skin caused by a sharp edge such as a knife or glass.* The wound edges are well defined and often straight, with little surrounding bruising.

Laceration *A breach in the skin caused by blunt force.* The wound is irregular with tearing of the tissues (Latin *lacerare*—to tear). This could be due to a fall, a blow from a blunt object, or a crushing force.

Contused wound *A breach in the skin with surrounding bruising.*

Penetrating wound *A wound with a fine path made by a pointed object.*

Contusion *An area of bruising due to blunt force, without a break in the skin.*

Haematoma *A subcutaneous collection of blood giving rise to a fluctuant swelling.*

Source: Critchley, M. (ed.) (1978). *Butterworths medical dictionary* (2nd edn). Butterworth, London.

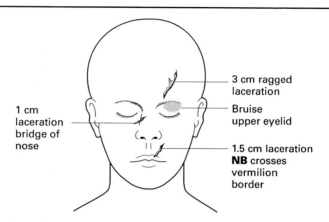

1 cm
laceration
bridge of
nose

3 cm ragged
laceration

Bruise
upper eyelid

1.5 cm laceration
NB crosses
vermilion
border

Fig. 1.4 • Example of a stamp for recording of wounds. The use of diagrams makes notes easier to understand.

Wound description

It is always better and quicker to *use diagrams* to show the position and type of wound. Many A&E departments make use of rubber stamps of various parts of the body which give an instant print of the appropriate part of the body (see Fig. 1.4).

If the wound is especially significant then *photography* should be considered. Polaroid photographs provide a permanent record of the original wound as well as reducing the number of wound inspections prior to definitive surgery.

Always try to *measure* wounds. A small flexible ruler is ideal.

Record the treatment (including the number of sutures).

> **Use correct words, measure wounds, use diagrams.**

References and further reading

1. Gilbert, F.J., Campbell, R.S.D., and Bayliss, A.P. (1990). The role of ultrasound in the detection of non-radiopaque foreign bodies. *Clinical Radiology*, **41**, 109–12.
2. Ginsberg, M.J., Ellis, G.L., and Flom, L.L. (1990). Detection of soft-tissue foreign bodies by plain radiography, xerography, computed tomography, and ultrasonography. *Annals of Emergency Medicine*, **19**, 701–3.
3. de Lacey, G., Evans, R., and Sandin, B. (1985). Penetrating injuries: how easy is it to see glass (and plastic) on radiographs? *British Journal of Radiology*, **58**, 27–30.
4. Knight, B. (1996). *Forensic pathology.* Edward Arnold/Hodder & Stoughton Educational, London.

CHAPTER 2

Initial management of life-threatening wounds

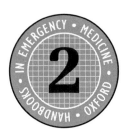

Serious penetrating wounds

- Introduction • Aetiology • Initial triage
- Unstable patient
- Circulation and haemorrhage control • Stable patient

Introduction

In the United Kingdom only 4 per cent of serious injury is due to penetrating trauma. However, all penetrating wounds of the trunk, neck, and face presenting to the A&E department must be regarded as serious. The size and appearance of the skin wound does not give a reliable indication of the severity of the deep damage.

> **Any shocked patient with a penetrating trunk wound requires immediate surgical referral with concurrent resuscitation.**

Assess these patients *rapidly* and *thoroughly*. Wounds of vital organs such as the heart can kill within minutes, but if they are treated quickly then the patient will have a good chance of survival.

If a patient with a penetrating trunk wound arrives in the A&E department in an unstable condition then the surgical team **must** be called **immediately**. These is much that the A&E department can do to commence resuscitation, but this is one situation where immediate surgical assistance can be dramatically life-saving, as in cases of cardiac tamponade or a cut femoral artery and vein.

This section will deal with penetrating wounds of the trunk as a whole. Remember that the upper abdomen and the lower chest are often both injured in wounds of the trunk. A stab wound anywhere between the nipples and the level of the umbilicus may involve both compartments (Fig. 2.1). A gunshot wound anywhere on the trunk may damage organs in both chest and abdomen.

Similarly wounds of the neck may involve the upper chest.

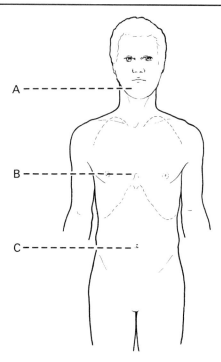

Fig. 2.1 . A stab wound between levels A and B may damage structures both in the neck and thorax. Between Levels B and C might damage structures both in the thorax and abdomen. A gun shot wound anywhere between A and C might damage structures in all 3 compartments.

Aetiology

In routine A&E work the commonest penetrating trunk injuries are *stab* wounds caused by assault. But penetrating injuries may also occur at work, for example in the mining and steel industries as a result of impacts from *high-speed metal fragments* from hammering or machinery. They may also occur in road traffic accidents as a result of objects coming into the cab or through the occupant's being ejected and *impaled*.

Gunshot wounds of the trunk are relatively uncommon in mainland UK. Gunshot wounds to the head are an often-used method of suicide.

Part of the injury complex seen following an *explosion* is due to penetration by debris of varying size. Such injuries are rare, but the presence of other types of injury (burns, inhalation injury, and blast injury) must be considered.

Initial triage

All penetrating trunk injuries are potentially serious, but the presence of ONE of the findings in Box 2.1 indicates that an immediate threat to life is present, and these patients should be classed as **unstable**.

Box 2.1 **Clinical indications of an unstable patient**

1. *Presence of clinical shock*
   The initial look at the patient's face and palpation of the pulse are the best clinical guides to the presence of shock. The pale, anxious, slightly confused facies, the cold clammy periphery, the fast and low-volume pulse signify 20 per cent to 30 per cent of total blood volume has been lost. In the elderly and in young children these signs may be manifest with a lower percentage loss.
   Blood pressure is a **very poor** indicator of initial, severe blood loss.
2. *Respiratory difficulty*
   Wounds of the face, jaws, or neck may cause upper-airway problems.
   Chest wounds may interfere with ventilation.
3. *Respiratory rate greater than 29 breaths per minute.*
4. *Respiratory rate less than 12 breaths per minute.*
   This indicates severe hypoventilation.
5. *Glasgow Coma Score less than 13.*
6. *Systolic blood pressure less than 90 mmHg.*

This list is by no means exhaustive. The history of the injury may well indicate a need for urgency and if there is any doubt then it is best to classify the patient as unstable and act accordingly (Fig. 2.2).

Unstable patient

Airway

If there is a possibility of airway injury then further help should be called immediately.

The life-threatening wounds are severe wounds of the face, such as open fractures of the mandible, or penetrating wounds of the neck.

Speed in securing the airway is essential, but it is often an extremely difficult situation. The patient may well be hypoxic, and thus thrashing around and unable to co-operate.

Unstable patient
Call surgeons

Airway	Breathing
Oxygen	Relieve tension pneumothorax
Suction	Chest drains if indicated
?ET tube	Cover sucking chest wounds
?Surgical airway	

Circulation	
Empty neck veins	*Full neck veins*
Place two large IV lines	?Tension pneumothorax
Blood for cross match	?Cardiac tamponade
Adequate IV fluid	
Immediate surgery	

Fig. 2.2 • Management of an unstable patient with a penetrating trunk wound.

Endotracheal intubation by a skilled A&E doctor or anaesthetist is the best method of securing the airway. A doctor should be standing by to proceed to a surgical airway if endotracheal intubation fails.

Surgical airway. Surgical cricothyroidotomy or needle cricothyroidotomy may be appropriate for facial wounds (see p. 185). Direct penetrating wounds of the larynx or trachea present difficulties in management, but emergency access may be gained by passing a tracheostomy tube through the wound into the trachea.

Breathing The immediately life-threatening conditions causing breathing difficulties are:

- tension pneumothorax
- a sucking chest wound
- massive haemothorax

Assess:

- the respiratory rate
- the presence of dyspnoea
- chest movement: unequal expansion is the best way to detect unilateral pneumothorax
- for tracheal deviation and dilated neck veins
- for percussion note and breath sounds

Treatment
Tension pneumothorax. This is a clinical diagnosis (see p. 187). Do not wait for X-ray confirmation. Insert a 16-gauge cannula into the second intercostal space in the mid-clavicular line. A chest drain is then inserted (see p. 191).

Sucking chest wounds are covered with occlusive dressings and a chest drain is inserted.

Massive haemothorax is treated by chest drainage, blood transfusion, and early surgery.

Circulation and haemorrhage control

Hypovolaemia due to blood loss is the commonest cause of shock in a penetrating trunk wound.

Tension pneumothorax and cardiac tamponade are rapidly lethal conditions which must be excluded in chest and upper abdominal wounds.

Assess
Look for the signs of shock (pallor, sweating, restlessness, cool clammy periphery).
Check capillary refill time (normally less than 2 seconds).
The pulse is often fast and low volume (beware: the pulse may be slow, especially in young and fit individuals and in those with profound hypovolaemia).
Check the neck veins, since venous distension in the presence of shock will indicate a tension pneumothorax or cardiac tamponade (obstructive shock).

Treatment
Hypovolaemic shock. Call the surgical team immediately. Secure venous access using at least two 16-gauge cannulae, and send blood for cross-matching. Request type-specific blood if there are any signs of shock, and O-negative blood if the patient is severely shocked.
   Apply direct pressure to any external haemorrhage.
   The shocked patient with a penetrating wound needs immediate surgical assessment. Immediate surgery to control haemorrhage is THE priority. The evidence suggests that high-volume fluid replacement carries a higher mortality than minimal fluids and early surgery.

The treatment of blood loss in penetrating trauma is early surgery.

Obstructive shock. Tension pneumothorax and cardiac tamponade both cause shock by reducing cardiac filling. The treatment of each condition is outlined elsewhere (see pp. 187 and 189), but rapid volume infusion is also indicated to increase right-heart filling pressure.

Stable patient

The primary survey will identify the patient who is fully alert with a clear airway, no trouble breathing, and no signs of shock.

Take time to assess the patient fully. Remember that injured patients may deteriorate very quickly, and watch constantly for any change in the clinical condition. The assessment must not be delayed, and the surgical team should be notified that such a patient is in the hospital (Fig. 2.3).

Even if the patient is stable, venous access should be secured at the earliest opportunity.

1. Take a full history and perform a thorough examination. Remember **look** at **the back**.
2. Chest X-ray is mandatory for penetrating wounds of the trunk.
3. In gunshot wounds the chest and abdominal X-rays will help plot the path of the missile.
4. An urgent IVP/contrast CT is indicated if renal damage is suspected.
5. The tetanus status should be ascertained and appropriate prophylaxis given.
6. Measure and record all wounds accurately. It is always possible that serious criminal charges will be involved, and your notes should be professional in content and accuracy.

Stable patient

Primary survey (**A**irway **B**reathing **C**irculation)
Undress FULLY
IV access
Full history
Secondary survey
Erect Chest X-ray (other X-ray)
Surgical opinion

Fig. 2.3 . Management of stable patient with penetrating trunk wound.

7. Refer and admit. In many cases there will be little doubt that the patient requires admission to hospital. There is a school of thought (mainly among inexperienced junior surgeons or in *very* experienced surgeons working in centres abroad dealing with large numbers of penetrating wounds) that such wounds may be adequately explored under local anaesthesia in the A&E department. Such a procedure should not be carried out by the A&E staff. The majority of these wounds will require admission to hospital for observation.

Serious blunt trauma

Wounds caused by serious blunt trauma are much more common than penetrating wounds in A&E practice in the United Kingdom.

Most patients with life-threatening blunt injury will have at least one wound. However it is not usually these wounds which pose the threat to life, but the damage to deeper structures due to the transmission of the forces of blunt violence. Wounds in this context are often important clues to the type and direction of the violence, indicating which internal structures are at risk.

The initial treatment and resuscitation of patients with blunt injury is a huge topic, and for further details of this subject the reader is referred to the book in this series entitled *The management of major trauma*. The principles are similar to those given above for resuscitation in cases involving penetrating wounds.

In the severely injured patient wounds may not have the highest priority, but it is essential that the basics of wound care are not forgotten. All wounds should be assessed and noted. Formal treatment may be delayed, but the wounds should be cleaned and dressed, and definite plans should be made for definitive treatment once life-threatening injuries have been treated. Tetanus prophylaxis is essential.

Further reading

1. Driscoll, P. (1996). Initial assessment and management. In *ABC of major trauma* (ed. D. Skinner, P. Driscoll, and R. Earlam) pp. 1–5. British Medical Journal Publications, London.
2. Robertson, C. and Redmond, A. (1994). *The management of major trauma*. Oxford University Press.
3. Bickell, W.H., Wall, M.J., Pepe, P.E., Martin, R.R., Ginger, V.F., Allen, M.K., and Mattox K.L. (1994). Immediate versus delayed fluid resuscitation for hypotensive patients with penetrating torso injuries. *New England Journal of Medicine*, **331**, 1105–9.

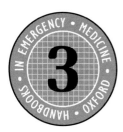

Legal aspects of wound care

Working in the A&E department is almost certainly going to bring the junior doctor into contact with the police and legal system, often for the first time. The police or solicitors may require patient details, either for criminal prosecutions in assault cases or civil actions in injury cases.

Records and notes

The medical notes made at the time of examination are extremely important legal documents. Full and accurate notes must be kept of all patient contacts. This is especially true in the patient with a wound. You may be called upon to write a police statement *many months* after having seen the patient.

You may be called to court, and your notes may be presented to the court; thus it is important that the notes are professional in content and presentation.

Review of notes by the patient

Since November 1991 any patient has the right to read his or her medical notes. This emphasizes the need to make clear and accurate notes, and to beware of making any 'funny' or pejorative remarks.

Medical negligence

Many doctors starting work in A&E are worried by the potential for litigation. It is true that there are a significant number of legal actions each year concerning A&E, but the chances of such an action are less than 1 in 10 000 cases.

Patient expectations are increasing dramatically. Complaints arise from the following areas of wound care:

- Failure to diagnose a foreign body, especially glass
- Failure to diagnose nerve/tendon/vessel damage

- Dissatisfaction with the cosmetic result
- Wound infection

Some of these errors are avoidable. Take X-rays in glass wounds, examine nerve/tendon function meticulously, and ensure every wound is properly cleaned. If you adhere to a good routine of accurate history and examination, appropriate investigations and treatment, AND KEEP GOOD NOTES, it is unlikely that you would be criticized successfully. Remember that common sense and good patient communication are also important in avoiding these problems.

Errors do happen, and the more patients that you see, the greater the chance of error. If you make a mistake then tell your consultant IMMEDIATELY. The sooner this is done, the sooner any necessary remedial action can be taken. To make a mistake is human but it is a mark of personal and professional maturity to admit such errors.

Police statements

There is usually no need to give a formal statement to the police immediately after the patient has been seen. Routine requests for such statements should be referred to the hospital administration. It is best to write the statement yourself. Beware of oral statements dictated to a policeman, since the wording may significantly alter the meaning of the statement.

The statement should be on a witness statement form (MG11), and a suggested format is given on p. 33.

Begin the statement by giving your full name, your qualifications, and how you came to be involved with the patient. You should then identify the person you examined by his or her full name and date of birth.

Although history is an important part of the medical examination, the description by the patient of the events leading to the injury is 'hearsay', and thus not admissible as evidence; however, you should give some indication of the mechanism of the injury, and list the patient's complaints and symptoms.

Keep to the facts, and avoid conjecture or expressing opinions that may be difficult to defend under cross-examination.

If there is more than one injury, list each of the injuries in turn, giving the findings on examination, the results of any X-rays, and any treatment given. Try to use words that a lay person will understand (if accurate anatomical descriptions are needed then put these in parentheses after the lay description). Give an indication if the patient is to be seen for follow-up of the injury.

The statement must be signed and dated at the top of the first page and at the bottom of EVERY page. These signatures MUST be witnessed.

Keep a copy of all statements given to the police. The statement can then be returned to the police with a form to claim the fee for the statement.

Sample police statement

STATEMENT OF WITNESS

STATEMENT OF   Dr Andrew Hamilton Black
DATE OF BIRTH 14.11.63
ADDRESS AND TELEPHONE NUMBER   Doctors Mess,
Blankshire DGH.
0000–3003000

This statement, consisting of . . . pages each signed by me, is true to the best of my knowledge and belief and I make it knowing that, if it is tendered in evidence, I shall be liable to prosecution if I have wilfully stated in it anything which I known to be false or do not believe to be true.

Dated the . . . . . . day of 1997

Signed . . . .
Signature witnessed by . . . .

I am Dr Andrew Hamilton Black, MB, ChB. On the night of Saturday 17 March 1997 I was on duty as Senior House Officer in the Accident and Emergency Department of the Blankshire District General Hospital.

History
At 23.40 hours on 17.3.97 I examined Mr Andrew White, date of birth ••.••.••.

He said that he had been assaulted and was complaining of pain in his right hand, jaw, and head.

He had not been unconscious.

Head
There was a deep 6 cm laceration on the back of the head (occiput), with some bleeding from this wound. Mr White was fully alert, and examination of the nervous system showed no sign of any damage to the brain.

The wound was cleaned, and under local anaesthetic three sutures were used to close the wound.

Face
There was bruising, swelling, and tenderness over the left side of the jaw. There was some bruising inside the mouth. There was no deformity and no damage to the teeth. X-ray showed no fractures.

No specific treatment was needed.

Right hand
There was swelling and tenderness over the knuckle of the little finger (neck of the little finger metacarpal). There was slight deformity of the metacarpal, with normal function of the tendons, nerves, and circulation. X-ray showed a slightly displaced fracture of the little finger metacarpal.

The finger and hand were placed in plaster of Paris and Mr White was instructed to keep the hand elevated. An appointment was made at the fracture clinic of this hospital on 19.3.97.

Mr White was given a supply of pain-killing tablets and

given instructions to return if there were problems due to his head injury or hand injury. He did not return.

Signed . . . . Signature witnessed by . . . .

Release of information to the police

The police may request the release of information without the consent of the patient.

The most common situation would be in a seriously injured patient who is unable to give consent. There is little doubt that all possible assistance should be given to the police in these circumstances. If a serious crime has been committed then it is most likely to be in the patient's best interests to co-operate with the police. If a relative is easily contactable then they may give consent.

Rarely, the police may request information on a patient whom they suspect of having committed a crime. The best course of action would be to refer the police to the consultant in charge of the department. For example, a burglar may have injured himself during the crime, and the police ask if the A&E register shows that this person has attended the department with an injury. The interests of the patient would not be served by giving the information to the police, and it is unlikely that the information would be released in these circumstances.

The 1972 Road Traffic Act requires the disclosure of the name and address of a driver involved in a road traffic accident, if they are alleged to be guilty of an offence under the Act. Again, such requests should be referred to the consultant in charge of the department.

When a serious crime has been committed then the doctor must weigh his or her responsibility to society with his or her responsibility to maintain confidentiality. If the crime is a serious arrestable offence, for example murder, attempted murder, manslaughter, or rape, then such information may be given. Such cases should be referred to the consultant.

If a terrorist crime is suspected then the information must be released.

Release of information to a third party

Accident and Emergency records belong to the Employing Authority of the doctor. In practice the Authority usually delegates the decision to release notes to the clinician in charge of the case. Records are usually freely available as long as no legal proceedings are envisaged against the Authority or its employees.

In most routine cases it is essential to have the *written consent* of the patient (or 'nearest friend', i.e. parent or guardian) before any details are released to a third party.

Medico-legal reports

These reports are requested by solicitors or insurance companies if a patient is pursuing a civil claim against another party who may be liable for damages. This may be a report from the records or may require a further examination of the patient.

Before providing any such report obtain the written consent of the patient and confirmation that no action is contemplated against the hospital or its employees (or you!).

The agency requesting the report will often ask for some indication of the prognosis, and this may be difficult for doctor with less than six months' experience in the A&E department.

Since January 1989 the patient has a right to see these reports before they are submitted to the requesting agency.

Such reports come with Category 2 of the Terms and Conditions of Service for hospital medical staff (work not directly related to patient care). The Crown Indemnity covering negligence claims arising from NHS clinical work does not cover such reports, and the basic subscription to the medical defence organizations does not automatically provide insurance. If you do intend to do such work check with your medical defence organization that you have the appropriate level of insurance cover.

Further reading

1. Montague, A. (1996). *Legal problems in emergency medicine.* Oxford University Press.
2. Touquet, R., Fothergill, J., and Harris, N. (1994). Accident and emergency departments; the speciality of accident and emergency medicine. In *Medical negligence* (ed. M. Powers and N. Harris) pp. 615–46 Butterworth, Sevenoaks, Kent.
3. Gee, D. and Mason, K. (1990). *The courts and the doctor.* Oxford University Press.
4. Knight, B. (1989). *Legal aspects of medical practice.* Churchill Livingstone, Edinburgh.

PART 2
Wound treatment

---

4 Anaesthesia

5 Surgical techniques of wound care

6 Wound infection

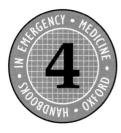

Anaesthesia

Choice of anaesthetic

Adequate wound examination and management is very difficult unless good analgesia and anaesthesia are achieved. The choice of anaesthetic will depend on many variables. An 'easy' eyelid wound in a strong, unreasoning three-year-old may be impossible to suture without general anaesthesia, while a large thigh wound may be very adequately treated using local techniques. If you foresee problems in obtaining adequate operating conditions using simple techniques, seek advice.

Local infiltration is the commonest anaesthetic technique in A&E wound care. It is simple and safe provided routine safety precautions are observed. Its use is limited by:

1. Over-large or too numerous wounds, which require large doses of anaesthetic.
2. Deep wounds requiring optimal conditions for the repair of deep structures (prolonged tourniquet use).
3. Patient factors, as with the toddler in whom local anaesthetic will still not provide good conditions for wound suture.

Distal nerve blocks, such as digital nerve blocks, wrist blocks, or ankle blocks, allow minor surgery on all the structures supplied by that nerve. Thus in a fingertip injury it is possible to shorten bone using a digital nerve block. The other great advantage is when it is difficult or even dangerous to inject the area around the wound directly: in the finger (even small volumes of anaesthetic can cause rises in tissue pressure); in infections (do not inject through an area of active infection); or in the sole of the foot (a tight tissue compartment makes the injection difficult and painful).

The disadvantages are that greater skill is required, the failure rate is higher, and there is a greater danger of complications, such as inadvertent intravascular injection or intraneural injection. However, the techniques are easily mastered given good training and supervision.

Proximal regional blocks, such as the axillary or supra-clavicular block, are used for complicated hand wounds.

These techniques require much greater skill and training. The doses of local anaesthetic used require that the doctor using such techniques should be available to monitor the patient throughout the procedure, and to treat any complications. They are not suitable for new junior staff in the A&E department.

General anaesthesia. This provides ideal conditions for wound care. It is mandatory for large, complicated, very contaminated wounds. It is also recommended in wounds requiring formal exploration (regional blocks are an alternative).

It will require an anaesthetist, anaesthetic and monitoring equipment, and a fasted patient.

Local anaesthesia in children

There is no 'best method' of providing anaesthesia for children's wounds. The choice of technique will depend on the type of wound, the attitude of the child, the parents' wishes, and individual department policy. This is a difficult area—do not be afraid to ask for advice.

General principles

The child should be offered analgesia *in triage* when appropriate. Discuss the management plan with the parents; their support is essential, and they will often be of great assistance in reassuring the child during the procedure. Explain carefully in language the child can understand. Never say 'it won't hurt' when you know it will, as you will lose the confidence of the child.

The help of one or two experienced nurses is vital. Distraction techniques (e.g. music) may be helpful in children of all ages. In some A&E departments play therapists or staff with special training may be available to provide distraction.

Restraint may be used in toddlers if the wound is small and the surgical procedure brief.

Tissue glue and skin closure strips These methods should be used whenever possible (see pp. 77 and 76).

Local anaesthesia This is used if the wound is not suitable for closure with tissue glue or skin closure strips. Ensure that the procedure can be performed without exceeding the safe maximum dose of local anaesthetic and within a reasonable time. It has been shown that warming lignocaine to 37 °C immediately before use reduces the pain of injection; buffering the lignocaine may also help. Always use the finest needle available and inject slowly. Allow sufficient time for the local anaesthetic to act.

Peripheral nerve blocks Consider using these when possible as they may reduce the number of injections and total volume of local anaesthetic required.

General anaesthesia May be necessary even with small wounds. Sometimes ideal surgical conditions are needed to achieve satisfactory results. Although general anaesthesia involves additional risks and may lead to treatment delay and perhaps hospital admission, there may be no other acceptable option.

Other options

Hypnosis. This is advocated by some as an effective means of reducing the pain of invasive procedures.

Topical local anaesthetic agents. TAC (tetracaine, adrenaline, and cocaine), cocaine, and LAT (lignocaine, adrenaline, and tetracaine), are commonly used in North America. EMLA® (lignocaine and prilocaine) is also effective. However, none of these preparations are licensed for use in the UK, although they are in fact used in some A&E departments.

Sedation. Oral midazolam has been shown to be safe and effective, but is not yet licensed for use in the UK. Intravenous midazolam may be used, but only by those with appropriate training. It is vital to monitor the ECG, respiratory rate, and SaO_2 when administering sedation.

Local anaesthetic agents

• **Lignocaine**   • **Complications**   • **Other agents**

Lignocaine

This is the most commonly used agent. It is very safe as long as certain precautions are observed:

1. Do not exceed the safe maximum does—3 mg/kg, which is 20 ml of 1 per cent plain lignocaine in a 70 kg patient. The dose may be increased by the use of adrenaline.
2. Ensure the patient is not allergic to local anaesthetics.
3. Use lower total doses on patients with epilepsy, hepatic impairment, cardiac conduction defects, and in elderly patients.
4. The use of lignocaine is contraindicated in porphyria, complete heart block, and hypovolaemia.
5. DO NOT USE LIGNOCAINE AND ADRENALINE SOLUTIONS IN THE HANDS, FEET, EARS, NOSE, OR PENIS. Use in these appendages results in ischaemia and possible loss of tissue.

Box 4.1 **Lignocaine use**

• Maximum safe dose 3 mg/kg, e.g. 70 kg adult—20 ml of 1% solution. 20 kg child—6 ml of 1% solution.
• Do not use lignocaine and adrenaline in hand, foot, nose, ears, or penis

---

The formulations available:

1 per cent solution is the most commonly used for infiltration anaesthesia.

0.5 per cent solution is used if the wound is large or there are many wounds.

2 per cent solution is used where small volumes are required, as in digital nerve blocks (**note**: total maximum does is 10 ml).

Lignocaine and 1:200000 adrenaline solutions may be OF OCCASIONAL USE in A&E work. In most departments these solutions are stored separately from the plain solutions, to minimize the chances of their inadvertent use on a finger. If adrenaline-containing solutions are used, then the total maximum dose is increased to 7 mg/kg (50 ml of 1 per cent solution in 70 kg adult).

Complications Overdosage with a local anaesthetic can cause death. Care is needed to ensure that intravascular injections are not given, and that the maximum total dose is not exceeded.

Box 4.2 **Early symptoms of lignocaine toxicity**
- Numbness of mouth and tongue
- A feeling of light-headedness
- Tinnitus

If these occur then stop the injection and assess the patient. The main danger is that convulsions may occur. Move the patient to a resuscitation area and secure venous access.

Give high-flow oxygen. If no further symptoms occur then observe the patients for 30 minutes. The early signs of local anaesthetic toxicity are similar to those of fainting or hyperventilation.

If the speech becomes slurred, or there are muscle twitchings or convulsions, then ask for senior help.

If convulsions do occur then the priority is to maintain adequate ventilation. Skilled assistance will be needed.

Diazepam 5–10 mg should be given intravenously to control convulsions.

If hypoxia and prolonged convulsions can be avoided, then adverse cardiac effects may not occur. Treat hypotension below 90 mmHg systolic with a 500 ml intravenous bolus of fluid.

Other agents

Bupivicaine (Marcain) is not routinely used in the care of wounds. The main advantage is the prolonged duration of anaesthesia of up to 8 hours which this agent gives. The disadvantage is that the onset of anaesthesia is delayed. It is of specific use where a procedure may be very painful after the operation. The maximum total dose is 60 ml of 0.25% solution.

Local infiltration

Use 0.5 or 1.0 per cent plain lignocaine.

Plan to perform injection well before commencing cleaning or suturing—the agents take time to work. The commonest reason for poor anaesthesia is failure to allow sufficient time for the anaesthetic to work!

Check the solution as you draw it up:

Is it the right solution?

What is the safe total dose?

Use an alcohol swab to clean AROUND the wound.

Figure 4.1 shows alternative techniques of local infiltration, either *through* the wound or by a field block *around* the wound.

If infiltrating through the wound edge, a series of small injections are given into the subcutaneous layer.

If performing a field block, commence at one end of the wound, slip the needle through the skin, and advance through the subcutaneous tissues. Inject the anaesthetic as the needle is withdrawn. Do not withdraw completely from the skin, but alter the angle and repeat at the other side of the wound. Approximately 1 ml is injected with each pass of the needle. If a second puncture is required always introduce the needle through previously anaesthetized skin.

Wash your hands, glove up, prepare the instruments, clean the wound, explore, and repair it.

IF the anaesthetic appears NOT to be working—allow more time!

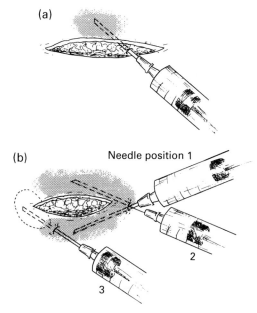

Fig. 4.1 . Techniques of local infiltration. (a) Through the wound edge.
(b) Field block: insert needle to one side of wound of tip of needle.
From same puncture site, infiltrate other side of wound. Reintroduce
needle through previously anaesthetized skin.

Finger blocks

Space is limited in the fingers, and it can be difficult to inject
anaesthetic solutions, especially on the volar surfaces.

Some form of nerve block is required. Various techniques
are described to block the digital nerves; the commonest
technique is a metacarpal head block by the dorsal approach
(Fig. 4.2).

> **PLAIN anaesthetic solutions are used. NO adrenaline
> should be used in the hand.**

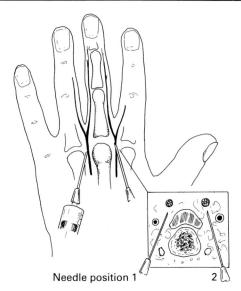

Needle position 1   2

Fig. 4.2 • Metacarpal head block—dorsal approach.

In performing a metacarpal head block 3–4 ml of 2 per cent plain lignocaine are used.

1. The hand is placed flat with the dorsum uppermost.

2. Using a blue (23-gauge) needle puncture the skin at the level of the base of the web and pass the needle to a position just proximal to the metacarpal head.

3. Aspirate to ensure the needle is not in a vessel, then inject 1 ml of lignocaine.

4. Draw back the needle and redirect it towards the palm, injecting 1 ml of lignocaine adjacent to the base of the proximal phalanx.

5. Repeat the procedure on the other side of the finger.

A digital nerve block aims to anaesthetize the digital nerves in the palm, where they lie beside the flexor tendons.

1. Locate the flexor tendon at the level of the distal palmar crease. The hand is laid flat with the palm upwards. Resisted flexion of the finger may make the tendon more easily palpable (Fig. 4.3).

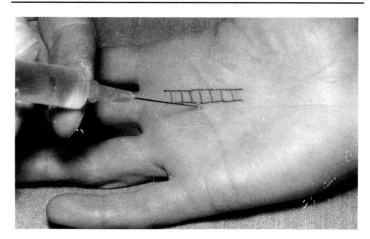

Fig. 4.3 • Digital nerve block at the level of palmar crease. The hatched area indicates flexor tendon.

2. With a finger on the tendon the needle is advanced into the palm just deep to the palmar aponeurosis (this is not deep).

3. 2 ml of solution are injected (if resistance to injection is felt, direct the needle slightly more to the side).

4. This process is repeated at the other side of the tendon.

5. If the wound is on the dorsum of the finger then a further 1 ml can be placed transversely across the dorsum of the finger at the base.

It may take 5–10 minutes for these blocks to work.

An alternative technique providing good anaesthesia is to inject the anaesthetic into the tendon sheath (NOT into the tendon). This technique may aid the diagnosis of a tendon injury; if there is a breach in the tendon sheath at the level of the laceration the anaesthetic will be seen to flow out of the wound.

The thumb may be anaesthetized by locating the tendon of flexor pollicis longus at the level of the proximal thumb crease. The digital nerves lie at the sides of the tendon at the level of the proximal crease.

Wrist blocks

● **Median nerve**   ● **Ulnar nerve**   ● **Radial nerve**

Median nerve block

The median nerve supplies the sensory innervation to the radial side of the palm, to the thumb, and to the index and middle fingers.

It can be anaesthetized just proximal to the wrist, where it lies on the ulnar aspect and deep to the tendon of flexor carpi radialis.

Do not use this block in patients with a history of carpal tunnel syndrome.

1. Use 4–6 ml of 1 per cent plain lignocaine.
2. Insert a blue (23-gauge) needle at right angles to the skin about 5 mm away from the ulnar side of flexor carpi radialis (Fig. 4.4).
3. The nerve may be located by eliciting paraesthesiae (the patient complains of tingling in the distribution of the nerve) by searching with the needle; but this is not always necessary.
4. If paraesthesiae are felt, withdraw the needle slightly and inject 4–6 ml of the solution. THE AIM IS TO INJECT AROUND THE NERVE, *NOT* INTO THE NERVE.

Ulnar nerve block

The ulnar nerve lies on the radial side of and deep to the tendon of flexor carpi ulnaris. The dorsal branch crosses from the volar to the dorsal aspect of the wrist about the level of the ulnar styloid.

1. Use a blue (23-gauge) needle and 3–5 ml of 1 per cent plain lignocaine.
2. Insert on the radial side of flexor carpi ulnaris.
3. Always aspirate prior to injection—remember the ulnar artery lies close by. Inject 3–4 ml of plain lignocaine (Fig. 4.5).
4. The dorsal branch is blocked by subcutaneous injection

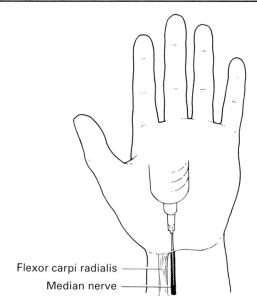

Flexor carpi radialis —
Median nerve —

Fig. 4.4 . Median nerve block.

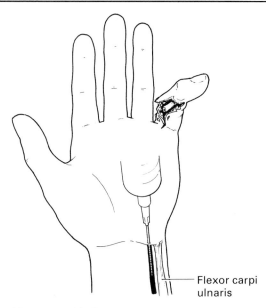

Flexor carpi
ulnaris

Fig. 4.5 . Ulnar nerve block.

of a further 3–5 ml of 1 per cent plain lignocaine over the ulnar side of the wrist.

Radial nerve block

The superficial radial nerve branches can be blocked by the subcutaneous injection of 4–5 ml of 1 per cent plain lignocaine around the radial border of the wrist.

Facial blocks

Ear block

This block is performed using 1.5 ml plain lignocaine. Insert the needle 1 ml below the earlobe and infiltrate subcutaneously on each side of the ear in a V-distribution (see Fig. 4.6). Aspirate prior to injection to ensure the needle is not in a vessel. Infiltrate to the level of the tragus anteriorly and to the level of the mastoid posteriorly. DO NOT USE ADRENALINE FOR THIS BLOCK.

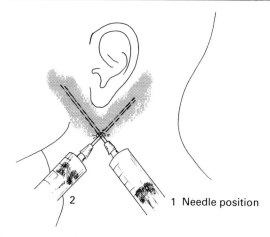

2   1 Needle position

Fig. 4.6 • Ear block. Infiltrate subcutaneously on each side of the ear in a V-distribution.

Forehead block

The supraorbital and supratrochlear nerves which supply the forehead may be blocked by local infiltration in a horizontal line commencing at the midline; 5 ml of 1 per cent lignocaine are required.

Ankle and foot blocks

Tibial and sural nerves

The skin of the sole is thick and tightly bound to the deep fascia. This makes local infiltration difficult and painful. By using ankle blocks these problems are overcome.

The tibial nerve supplies the distal part of the sole. It may be anaesthetized behind the medial malleolus.

1. The patient should lie prone with a pillow under the ankles.
2. The needle is inserted at the level of the upper border of the medial malleolus and just lateral to the posterior tibial pulse.
3. Inject 5–10 ml of 1 per cent plain lignocaine.

The sural nerve lies lateral to the Achilles tendon. Use 5 ml of 1 per cent plain lignocaine to infiltrate the subcutaneous tissues lateral to the Achilles tendon.

Further reading

1. Illingworth, K. A. and Simpson, K. (1998). *Anaesthesia and analgesia in emergency medicine.* Oxford University Press.
2. Trott, A. (1991). *Wounds and lacerations: Emergency care and closure.* Mosby, St. Louis, MO.
3. Gleeson, A. P. and Gray, A. J. (1995). Management of retained ear-rings using an ear block. *Journal of Accident and Emergency Medicine,* **12**, 199–201.
4. British Association for Accident and Emergency Medicine (1997). *Guidelines for Analgesia in Children in the Accident and Emergency Department.* BAAEM, London.

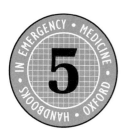

CHAPTER 5

Surgical techniques of wound care

Key points in surgical techniques

1 Give yourself the best possible operating conditions.

2 Ensure adequate anaesthesia.

3 Wound cleaning is THE most important part of wound care.

4 Examine the wound closely to exclude foreign bodies or damage to deep structures.

5 Consider the best method of wound closure—

    primary suture in most wounds.

    delayed primary closure in dirty wounds.

    adhesive tape closure in flap lacerations.

    glue in children and scalp wounds.

    excision and grafting—ask senior advice.

    leaving the wound to heal by granulation.

6 Approximate tissues without tension.

7 Having problems?

    Consider: better light

                better instruments

                an assistant

                senior help

Wound healing

The basic steps in wound healing are:

1. An acute inflammatory response. Results in the release of a protein-rich exudate into the wound. Fibrinogen results in coagulation of the exudate. White blood cells, including phagocytes, enter the wound to engulf dead cells.
2. Granulation tissue is formed by the ingrowth of capillaries and lymphatic vessels into the wound.
3. Epithelial cells regenerate from the margins of the wound and rapidly grow over the wound.
4. Fibroblasts and collagen fibres appear and the initial random process becomes organized.
5. The fibrous tissue matures into the wound scar, and the blood vessels become less obvious.

Factors altering wound healing

The speed at which healing takes place is variable and depends on:

(i) the site—some areas, such as the shin, always take longer to heal.

(ii) the blood supply—the rich vascular supply of the face usually ensures speedy healing.

(iii) movement in the scar—a wound over a joint, especially over the extensor surfaces, will take longer to heal.

(iv) closure technique—good technique with careful tissue handling are the keys to success in wound management.

(v) the wound configuration—tidy or untidy.

(vi) the cause of the wound—incised wounds heal better than crush injuries.

(vii) delay in management—this is a potent cause of infection leading to interruption of the healing process.

(viii) general factors:
- nutritional status—vitamin C and zinc deficiencies are specific deficits leading to poor wound healing, but general undernutrition will also delay healing
- age—a number of adverse factors operate to delay

healing in the elderly, such as peripheral vascular disease and capillary fragility
- diabetes mellitus
- steroid therapy
- irradiation/cytotoxic therapy

Few of the above factors can be influenced by the attending doctor, but those which can be—technique and the treatment of infection—are vitally important. Furthermore, an awareness of the above problems should alert the doctor to take increased care of a patient with these adverse factors.

Instruments and operating conditions
Requirements

To achieve a good result in the management of wounds the following conditions should be met:

1. A competent relaxed operator—it is essential that you are confident in the basic handling of instruments, basic suture technique, and knot-tying. Practice these skills in simulation (a cut in orthofelt does not scream!). A confident manner in the operator makes the patient feel at ease. If you can carry out a 'normal' social conversation it will help the patient relax and make the job much easier (distraction).
2. A comfortable patient who is confident in the operator— it is always advisable to have patients lying down to perform suturing. A sudden faint may well result in another wound to suture.
3. Adequate anaesthesia—a prerequisite to ensure wound cleaning and accurate closure.
4. Good illumination—peering into a dark hole will not lead to an accurate assessment of deep damage.
5. Satisfactory instruments—it is unfortunate that the instruments given to A&E departments are often less than adequate. The minimum requirements are: needle-holder, dissecting forceps (toothed), good sharp scissors, and small artery forceps. Every department should have packs available with finer instruments, including fine-toothed/non-toothed forceps, fine curved dissecting scissors, skin hooks,

and a small retractor. This makes the care of significant hand and facial wounds MUCH easier.

6. The correct suture and needle for the procedure.

Suture

The type of suture used will depend on the site and depth of the wound.

Absorbable sutures are used to approximate the deeper layers in a wound. They may also be used to approximate the skin in scalp lacerations and on fingertip injuries.

Vicryl® is the most commonly used absorbable suture. It is a synthetic braided material that handles well and holds knots. It retains 50 per cent of its tensile strength for 21 days. This can be a problem if used for surface closure as patients often return saying their sutures 'have not fallen out'. Vicryl Rapid® is more speedily absorbed.

Plain and chromic catgut are biological sutures. Chromic catgut retains 50 per cent of its tensile strength for up to 15 days. The tissue reaction is greater than with the synthetic materials.

Non-absorbable sutures are used for most skin closures. *Nylon* sutures tend to cause less tissue reaction and scarring, but handling may be more difficult, especially with monofilament nylon. The knots tend to slip more easily. *Silk* handles well and is much more 'forgiving' of suboptimal technique, but leaves more obvious scarring.

Suture gauge There is some confusion over the system used to describe the thickness of surgical sutures. The *metric number* of the suture is the diameter of the suture in millimetres multiplied by 10 (i.e. a 1 metric suture has a diameter of 0.1 millimetres).

The traditional *empirical gauge* system is still in widespread use to describe suture gauge.

Sutures of gauge 2/0 (3 metric) would be used in scalp lacerations, finer 4/0 (1.5 metric) sutures in hand cuts, and 5/0 or 6/0 (0.7 metric) sutures on facial wounds.

Note, however, that a thicker gauge of suture means a greater amount of foreign body and greater scarring. An inappropriately thick suture will result in more tissue disruption and local necrosis.

Needle

Different types and sizes of needle are available.

Round-bodied needles cause minimal tissue trauma, but do not penetrate skin well, and are not recommended, except for the closure of subcutaneous fat.

Reversed cutting and cutting needles are most commonly used in routine A&E work. Both are triangular in cross-section to ease tissue penetration. The difference is that the reversed cutting needle has its greater cross-section on the INSIDE of the curve of the needle. This makes the needle stronger and less likely to bend.

The choice of size depends on the 'bite' of tissue required. In general terms the deeper the wound the larger the needle required. Of course a deep wound may require layered closure, and in this case a small needle may be appropriate for the skin.

Box 5.1 Conditions for wound care
- Comfortable patient and operator
- Good light and instruments
- Good anaesthesia
- Assistance
- Correct needle and suture

Wound cleaning

• **Principles**   • **Cleaning solutions**   • **Methods**

Box 5.2 Principles of cleaning

THE best method of preventing wound infection is thorough wound cleaning. Any wound presenting to the A&E department must be regarded as contaminated.

The best time to ensure that all foreign material has been removed is at the time of initial presentation. If you find this impossible seek senior advice.

Adequate analgesia is needed. Usually local anaesthetic will suffice, but some wounds require general anaesthesia.

Social cleaning. Many injuries are sustained in less than ideal circumstances! It may be necessary to apply a small dressing to the wound and allow the patient to clean the surrounding areas. Soap and water are usually adequate, but degreasing agents such as Swarfega® should be available to be used to remove oil and grease.

Cleaning solutions

The commonly used solutions are:

(1) chlorhexidine
(2) normal saline
(3) iodine
(4) Savlon® and Tisept®
(5) tap water

Chlorhexidine may be spirit- or water-based; the former is more effective.

Iodine is most commonly used as povidone iodine (Betadine®). This may be spirit- or water-based. It may be used safely even when there is a history of iodine sensitivity.

Aqueous chlorhexidine and cetrimide solutions (Savlon®. Tisept®) are commonly used. They are less irritant to the tissues, but possibly less effective.

Tap water has been shown to be a safe wound cleaning agent and has the advantage that large volumes are readily available at no cost. Many studies have shown that the most important factor in preventing infection is the *volume* rather than the *type* of fluid used to clean the wound.

Methods

Aseptic technique is required for the protection of both the patient and the operator. It is best to use a 'clean' operating area (e.g. not that used for the incision and drainage of abscesses). The operator should wash his or her hands and use gloves. An apron and glasses may be needed if there is brisk bleeding or if copious lavage is required.

The area around the wound is cleaned using gauze swabs. Begin cleaning around the wound and move out to the periphery in a radial fashion.

Hold the edges of the wound apart and use the gauze swabs to remove clot, debris, and any other foreign material. This may cause bleeding, but direct pressure on the wound margins will allow inspection to ensure all material has been removed.

If the dirt is ingrained (as for example in a 'gravel graze') scrubbing with a scrubbing brush (or a sterile toothbrush for small wounds) may be needed. Adequate anaesthesia is essential.

Some very adherent material in the wound may need to be excised with scissors or scalpel.

Necrotic tissue should be excised, but there is no need to excise the wound widely, especially on the face and the volar surfaces of the fingers and palm.

The wound may then be irrigated with normal saline. Use a 20 ml syringe, and wash out the wound thoroughly. It cannot be overemphasized that cleaning and preparation of the wound is the key to the prevention of wound infection and good wound care, and the methods are summarized in Figure 5.1.

If it is not clean—do not close it!

Very deep wounds The deeper the wound the more difficult it will be to clean adequately, explore, and suture without general anaesthesia. It will also be more likely that deep structures will be damaged. Such wounds will need senior advice and optimal facilities for closure.

Thorough cleaning and haemostasis are essential to allow full inspection of the important structures near the wound. Any tendons exposed within a wound should be seen to go through their full range of movement in order to detect partial divisions (see p. 157). Any divided tendons, nerves, or large vessels will require repair.

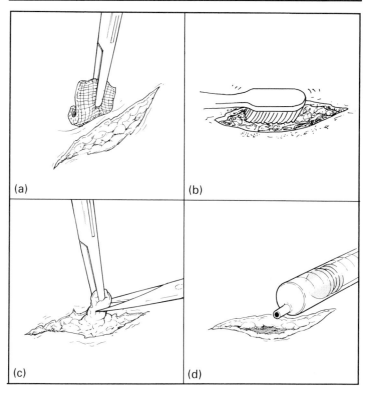

(a)

(b)

(c)

(d)

Fig. 5.1 . Methods of wound cleaning. (a) Antiseptic-soaked gauze swab to remove clot, debris, and foreign material. (b) Scrubbing to remove gravel. (c) Sharp dissection of heavily contaminated/non-viable tissue. (d) Saline lavage.

Wound examination

An essential part of wound care is adequate examination. This requires good anaesthesia, good light, and adequate haemostasis. The whole depth of the wound should be examined to ensure no deep structures are damaged. If difficulties are experienced they are commonly due either to inadequate anaesthesia, or bleeding obscuring the field. (See

Chapter 4 for details of anaesthetic techniques. See p.80 for control of bleeding). It is a common mistake to omit this stage of wound care, but the risk of missing deep structure damage is significant.

If suturing is to be delegated (e.g. to a nurse or medical student), it remains the responsibility of the doctor to examine the wound and rule out damage to deep structures. However in some departments trained nurse practitioners will take full responsibility for wound examination and management.

At times ideal conditions are impossible to achieve in a busy A&E department. If you think there may be significant deep damage, and the conditions for wound examination are not ideal, then it is best to refer to the in-patient team. Similarly, evidence of damage to tendons, nerves, or large vessels indicates the need for specialist advice and formal wound exploration in the operating theatre.

Technique

Wounds heal across their axis, and usually there is no contraindication to extending the wound in its long axis to achieve adequate exposure. THIS DOES NOT APPLY TO WOUNDS ON THE VOLAR SURFACES OF THE PALM AND FINGERS.

The main problem encountered is that of bleeding. An assistant is essential. All bleeding can be controlled by pressure on the wound margins. Adequate retraction is also essential if the wound is to be examined fully. You are not an octopus—get help! (Fig. 5.2).

A tourniquet can be of great help, but great care and discipline is needed to avoid limb-threatening ischaemic complications. See pp. 157 and 161 for a detailed description of tourniquet technique.

Principles of wound closure

The aim of primary closure of a wound is to approximate the wound edges accurately. This will speed the time to

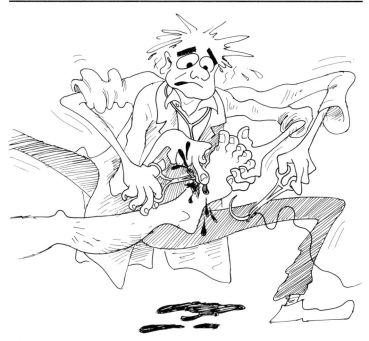

Fig. 5.2 . You are not an octopus! You cannot do everything, *get help.*

epithelial covering over of the defect, and will lead to a thinner wedge of scar tissue, and thus a better cosmetic result.

As in all medical interventions, these potential gains are at the cost of potential complications and problems:

1. Placing a suture will leave another scar in the suture track. This can be minimized by leaving the sutures for a minimum time, by avoidance of tying the suture too tight, and by avoiding infection.

2. Closing a wound which is not clean will result in wound infection, which will usually mean a worse scar and a potential for life-threatening infection.

3. Closure of the skin leaving a large 'dead space' will lead to haematoma, infection, and wound breakdown.

4. Placing sutures may interfere with blood supply and increase the risk of skin necrosis, especially in flap wounds and in areas of already precarious blood supply.

Primary closure by suture is the commonest method of wound closure practised in most A&E departments, and is safe provided the possible complications are kept in mind. Given good judgement and good technique the outcome is usually excellent.

Skin closure by interrupted suture
The instruments

Figure 5.3 shows the correct method of holding surgical instruments such as a needle-holder. The thumb and ring finger are used, with the index finger resting on the pivot of the instrument.

Toothed dissecting forceps are recommended in most skin suturing. They must be used with care or they will crush and tear the skin. Where the skin is thin or delicate (e.g. facial skin, the elderly) use skin hooks or non-toothed forceps.

The needle is held as shown in Figure 5.3. It must NOT be held near the end, or it will bend and possibly break in the tissues.

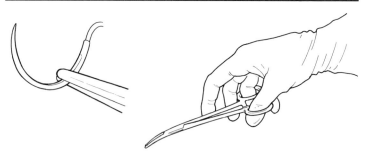

Fig. 5.3 • How to hold the needle and surgical instrument. The needle is held near the middle. The instrument is held with the thumb and ring finger.

Where do I start?

In most wounds there are 'clues' which help match the edges accurately. There may be a prominent skin crease, a small irregularity in the wound, or some other mark which will allow accurate apposition.

If there are no such aids then place skin hooks at either end of the wound and pull the wound closed. This will show the correct way to close the wound. Place one suture somewhere near the middle of the wound, and observe how the wound 'comes together' when this has been tied. If this does not 'look right' then cut the suture and try again. See Figure 5.4.

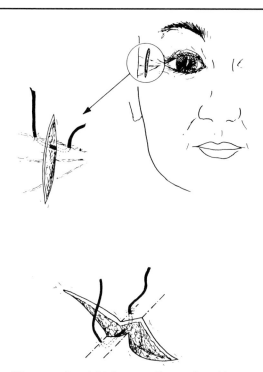

Fig. 5.4 . Where to place initial suture. Try to align skin creases or any irregularities in the wound edge. If it is difficult to see any line marks apply traction in the longitudinal axis of the wound—this should make the wound edges come together.

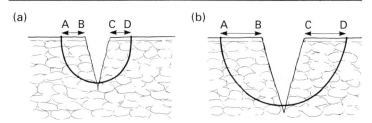

Fig. 5.5 . Distance from needle entry/exit points to wound edge. The greater the distance from the wound edge to the needle entry point, the deeper the bite of the needle. AB must equal CD, otherwise a step will occur.

How far from the wound do I puncture the skin?

Using curved needles, the further the distance from the edge of the wound, the deeper the 'bite' of the suture. If the wound is shallow, puncture the skin relatively close the skin edge.

Conversely, a deeper wound will require a larger bite, and the puncture point will be further from the wound (Fig. 5.5). If the wound is very deep a layered closure may be needed.

The skin edge is everted using forceps. The needle should enter at 90° to the skin.

How deep does the suture go?

The aim is to close the wound completely, leaving no dead space. If there are important structures immediately deep to the wound it is permissible to take the suture just to the deepest part of the wound (Fig. 5.6). If there are no important structures adjacent then carry the suture deep to the wound (Fig. 5.6).

How far from the wound does the needle emerge?

The needle should exit the skin at the same distance from the wound as it entered (Fig. 5.5, distance A–B = C–D). Failure to do this will lead to a 'step' in the wound when the suture is tied.

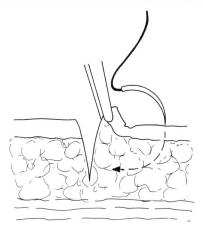

Fig. 5.6 • Depth of suture. Aim to close the wound fully by placing the suture to the deepest part of the wound. During needle insertion, the skin edges are everted by holding the subcutaneous tissues just below the skin edge with forceps or a skin hook. Ensure that the needle enters the skin at 90°.

How do I tie the knot?

This procedure is best taught by an experienced colleague using a simulated wound. Any material will do to practise knots.

Instrument ties are the easiest to master. Once the suture has been placed pull the material through to leave a short 'tail' (not too short, or you will pull the suture out).

Assume the suture has been placed from right to left across the wound (Fig. 5.7):

1. Take the *suture* in the left hand with the *needle-holder* in the right (Figure 5.7—'starting position').
2. Move the hands towards each other. The needle-holder lies against the suture. Wrap the suture over and around the instrument. Wrap it around again (Fig. 5.8).
3. Take hold of the end of the suture with the jaws of the needle-holder (Fig. 5.9).
4. Pull this first 'throw' down. The left hand goes to the right

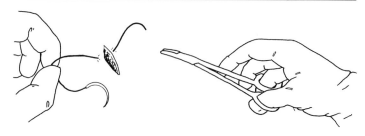

Fig. 5.7 • Instrument tie knot. Starting position, suture in left hand, needle-holder in right hand.

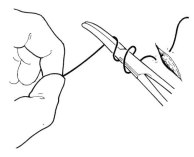

Fig. 5.8 • Wrapping the suture around the needle-holder. Do this TWICE.

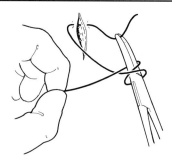

Fig. 5.9 • The first throw: take the loose end of the suture in the jaws of the needle-holder.

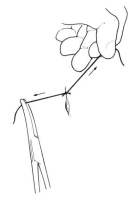

Fig. 5.10 . To tighten the first throw, cross the hands, needle-holder going to the left, and the left hand going to the right.

and vice versa (cross the hands). The knot should now lie 'flat'. Pull the suture to APPROXIMATE the tissues.

5. Let the end of the suture go. The 'short end' should now lie to the LEFT with the knot flat across the wound (Fig. 5.10).

6. Release the end of the suture, but keep the needle-holder in the same position over the wound (i.e. the hands are still crossed).

7. The left hand, still holding the suture is brought across to the left (as if to uncross the hands). This will bring the suture against the needle-holder. Wrap the suture around the needle ONCE.

8. Take hold of the 'short end' with the needle-holder.

9. Pull this second 'throw' down onto the first. The left hand pulls to the left, the right to the right. (Fig. 5.11). The knot should now 'lie' squarely.

10. Put at least one further 'throw' on the knot.

11. Cut the suture at 0.5 cm from the wound. Take care with nylon, which will tend to slip—leave longer.

Problems

If the tissues are springing apart, putting three 'throws' on the first knot may solve the problem. Alternatively, the first 'throw' of the suture may be 'locked'. To do this, at the stage

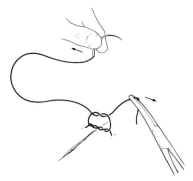

Fig. 5.11 • The second throw: the suture has been wrapped over the needle-holder in the opposite direction and this time the hand does not cross when tying the suture.

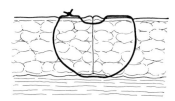

Fig. 5.12 • Mattress suture: after the first deep bite, the sutures returned through the skin edges to give better eversion and more accurate apposition.

of pulling the first throw down (Fig. 5.9) approximate the tissues as described by pulling to the left with the right hand and to the right with the left hand.

Once the correct tension is achieved uncross the hands, and this will lock the stitch.

Mattress suture

If the initial bite is deep a mattress suture may be used, to allow more accurate apposition and to evert the skin edges. The initial bite is placed as above, but the suture is returned, taking a small bite of the skin edge (Fig. 5.12). This suture should not be used on the face.

Layered closure

This method is probably UNDERUSED in wound closure in the A&E department. Failure to close deep layers will result in poor healing and increased complications.

Layered closure can also be used on moderately deep wounds where the cosmetic effect is important. Placing an accurate deep layer of sutures will allow the use of very small skin sutures or adhesive paper skin closures.

Absorbable suture material, such as Vicryl®, is used.

The sutures are inserted as shown in Figure 5.13. The first bite is taken UPWARDS through one side of the wound, and then the second bite is taken in a DOWNWARDS direction on the other side. This will 'bury' the knot, reducing the risk of sinus formation.

Suture removal

Once the wound has been treated the patient should be given instructions regarding further care.

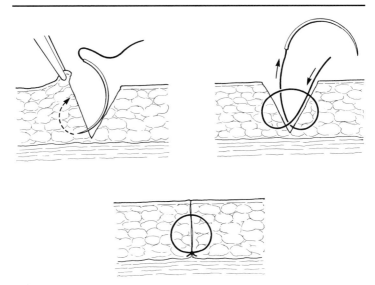

Fig. 5.13 • Layered closure: use this method to bury the knot for deep layers.

The wound should be kept clean and dry for at least 48 hours after primary suture. This will allow epithelial cover across the wound.

Patients should be told that if the wound is increasingly painful, or if there is spreading redness around the wound, they should return immediately.

The sutures will require removal. For many uncomplicated wounds the sutures may be removed by the patient's general practitioner or the practice nurse. If this is planned then give the patient a letter to inform the GP of the nature of the wound, the number of sutures, and the recommended date of removal.

The date of removal will depend on the position of the wound and the type of wound. Wounds over the extensor surfaces of joints, such as the fingers and knee, require at least 14 days before removal.

Box 5.3 Summary of wound suture and removal

Area	Suture	Removal
Face	6/0 nylon	4–5 days
Scalp	2/0 silk/nylon	7–10 days
Hands (non-extensor)	4/0 nylon	10 days
Hands (extensor surfaces)	4/0 nylon	14 days
Lower legs/feet	3/0–4/0 nylon	14 days
Other		7–21 days

Skin closure strips ('Steristrips')

These paper adhesive strips are widely used in A&E departments. They are less painful to apply, are less likely to cause tissue ischaemia, and save time. They are very useful in:

- children
- flap lacerations, especially in pre-tibial lacerations in the elderly

- some finger injuries—take care not to place circumferentially around a finger
- skin closure in wounds where a deep layer of sutures has approximated the skin edges

However, make sure that they are not used as a 'short cut' in wound care. It is essential that proper wound cleaning and exploration are carried out. Steristrips should not be applied over joints.

Strips are also difficult to use where there is much movement across the wound, as on the extensor surfaces of joints, on hairy skin, or where the skin is oily. Various types of product are available, including elasticated strips which may provide better closure where there is some skin movement.

Technique

Ensure full wound cleaning has been carried out. The surrounding skin must be DRY, so good haemostasis is important.

Adhesion to the skin may be increased by applying Tincture Benz Co. around the wound and allowing this to dry.

Place the 'long end' of the strip to one side of the wound, and, using tissue forceps, approximate the edges, and place the strip across the wound (Fig. 5.14).

If adhesion is a problem a further strip can be placed at right angles across the other strips.

Tissue glue (Histoacryl®)

The use of 'superglue' is a relatively recent but very useful addition to the methods of wound closure used in A&E. The principle is to bring the wound edges together and to use the glue to 'weld' the surface of the wound. See Figure 5.15. THE GLUE IS NOT PLACED INTO THE WOUND. If glue is placed in the wound it acts as a foreign body and the wound will not heal.

The glue is expensive, but a small amount may be with-

(a)

(b)

(c)

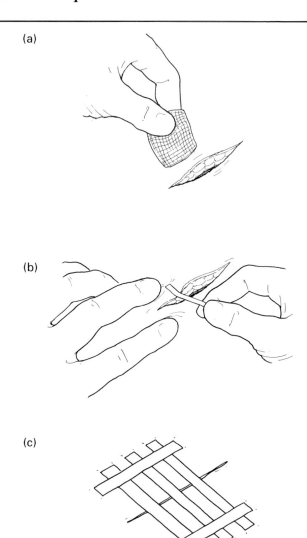

Fig. 5.14 • 'Steristrip' skin closure. (a) Apply tinc. benz co. around the area of the wound and allow to dry. (b) Apply Steristrip to one edge of the wound and bring the wound together. (c) Place further strips parallel to the wound to increase adhesion.

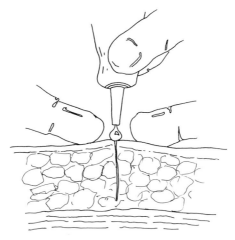

Fig. 5.15 . Technique of gluing. The skin edges are opposed and the glue is put onto the surface of the wound. Do not place glue INTO the wound.

drawn by sterile technique using a needle and syringe or sterile capillary tubing. The container may be resealed.

It is very useful in small cuts and lacerations in children. Take care around the eyes. Do not use on eyelids!

Technique

Clean the wound and achieve good haemostasis. Hold the wound edges together and place the glue along the wound either by a 'spot welding' technique or in a continuous line.

Hold the edges together for at least 30 seconds after application to allow the glue to polymerize and 'set'.

Staples

The use of skin staples for traumatic wounds has been shown to be an acceptable alternative to sutures. They may be quicker to apply. However, they only oppose the skin edges and are not suitable for deep wounds unless they are part of a layered closure. They require a special instrument to allow easy removal and this may limit their use as many patients are referred to GPs for suture removal.

Problem wounds

- Uncontrolled bleeding • Dirty wounds
- Deep wounds • Wounds under tension
- Untidy wounds

Uncontrolled bleeding

Proper wound management is impossible if blood fills the area! There is little point in inserting sutures blindly to control deep bleeding or to close the wound over active deep bleeding.

1. Get help—assistance is often in short supply, but another pair of hands will often solve the problem. If the bleeding is severe then ask for senior assistance, and apply direct pressure until help arrives.

2. Would better instruments help? Many suture packs are less than ideal. Ask for good instruments, and ensure that a plentiful supply of swabs is available.

3. Is the lighting sufficient?

4. Don't panic!

5. Ask the assistant to press on the wound edges, with just enough pressure to stop the bleeding. ALL bleeding stops with direct pressure. This should allow identification and control of any bleeding point.

6. In the limbs a tourniquet may be of great value (see p. 157 for details of use).

7. Small vessels, especially veins, may require ligation. Localized bleeding points may be undersewn (Figure 5.16). Do not take large bites of tissue in the hope of controlling bleeding. This will often fail, and may damage associated structures.

8. If a large 'named' artery (radial, ulnar, etc.) is the cause of the bleeding, ask for help. Such vessels will require microvascular repair.

If all the above have failed—apply firm pressure and get help.

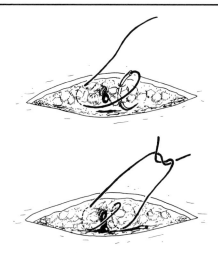

Fig. 5.16 . Undersewing of bleeding vessels.

Dirty wounds

The only time to clean a wound is at the initial presentation. All dirt should be removed. If this is not done the chance of wound infection is much increased.

> Box 5.4 **Any dirt in the superficial layers which is not removed at time of presentation will remain permanently in the wound as a type of tattoo.**

Adequate analgesia is essential.

Where wounds are very dirty, deep, and irregular, especially where there is much soil contamination, meticulous cleaning is essential. This may require general anaesthesia. In children with large dirty facial wounds general anaesthesia is always desirable for wound cleaning.

Good light, good instruments, and assistance are invaluable.

Techniques

Simple removal. Use forceps to pick out the fragments.

Sharp dissection. Use when the fragments are very adherent to the tissues. Small sharp scissors are the best 'weapon' to use. Non-viable tissue should also be excised by sharp dissection. Leaving non-viable tissue in the depths of the wound may cause clostridial infection.

Scrubbing. This is very effective in dirty grazes. A scrubbing brush (or a sterile toothbrush) is used.

Irrigation. This is essential in all dirty wounds. Once all obvious contamination is removed use large volumes of saline to wash out the wound. Povidone iodine may be used.

Delayed primary closure. If wounds are heavily contaminated the following technique is strongly advised:

1 Clean and examine the wound.
2 Sutures *may* be placed, but the ends are left long and untied, and the wound is packed with an antiseptic dressing (e.g. saline gauze or antibiotic impregnated paraffin gauze).
3 The patient is seen at daily intervals and the pack is replaced. At between 2 and 4 days, if the wound appears uninfected, the sutures may be tied.

Secondary closure. High-velocity bullet wounds, war wounds, and wounds where there is much tissue destruction are left widely open and are dressed for up to 14 days, when secondary suture may be performed if the wound is clean.

Deep wounds

The deeper the wound the more difficult it is to manage without proper general or regional anaesthesia. There is a greater chance that important deep structures will be damaged. A senior opinion is essential.

Detailed exploration is essential. This may require significant wound extension. Full haemostasis must be achieved to prevent deep haematoma.

Each layer is carefully cleaned. Contaminants often lie hidden in the depths. Any damage to deep structures will require immediate repair, so refer for appropriate senior advice.

A layered closure will be needed (see p. 75). A drain is not normally required, but use small vacuum drains if necessary.

Wounds under tension

If there has been some tissue loss, either during the initial accident or during subsequent cleaning, it may not be possible to oppose the skin edges without undue tension. Pulling the suture tight will either tear the skin or render the skin ischaemic and result in necrosis.

Undermining the wound can mobilize the skin to allow adequate closure (Fig. 5.17). The connective tissues attaching the skin to underlying structures are dissected clear. Great care must be taken to ensure that the blood supply to the flaps and wound margins is not compromised.

If undermining is not possible or fails to achieve closure without tension then seek senior advice. It may be acceptable to perform a partial closure and to allow the defect to heal by granulation.

In cosmetically important areas like the face or hands, primary closure is particularly important, and other techniques, such as skin flaps or skin grafts, may be required. Any facial wound that cannot be closed primarily should be referred immediately to plastic surgery.

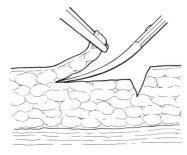

Fig. 5.17 . Undermining of skin flap.

Untidy wounds

Traumatic wounds come in all shapes and sizes, and by definition are not planned to enable easy closure! There may be skin flaps, extensions away from the main wound, or some skin loss.

Skin flaps present potential problems with ischaemia, therefore do not place too many sutures.

In complex wounds, close the main wound first, and then close any side extensions.

If partial closure is made necessary then leave the side extensions open, rather than the main wound.

If the wound edges are of unequal thickness, always place the knot on the thickest side.

Wound dressing

- **Closed wounds** • **Open wounds** • **Necrotic wounds**
- **Infected wounds** • **Sloughy wounds**
- **Granulating wounds** • **Epithelializing wounds**

There is a great growth industry in the many different wound coverings available. Dressings are of two main types, those for wound covering, and those involved in managing untidy or infected wounds.

No single dressing is suitable for all wounds nor at all times during the healing process. The selection depends on:

- the size and type of wound
- the frequency of change of dressing
- patient comfort and ease of removal
- the overall cost of management

Each department will have routine wound dressings for each category of wound. Advice of experienced A&E staff, either nursing or medical, is invaluable in the choice of the appropriate dressing.

Closed wounds

There is no good evidence that dressing a sutured wound will reduce the risk of wound infection. However, in treating out-patients it is probably best to apply a light dressing of non-adherent gauze. This will absorb any exudate and stop irritation of the wound by clothing. It may also remind the patient not to manure the garden or clean the septic tank!

If it is desirable to observe the wound then the transparent dressing Opsite may be used. This dressing is semipermeable and adhesive, but impermeable to bacteria.

Open wounds

Types of wound dressings available for the management of open wounds are listed in Table 5.1. The aim is to encourage clean granulation tissue by providing a moist environment free from slough.

Necrotic wounds

Surgical excision is the best method of removing dehydrated dead epithelium. If this is not practical then reversing dehydration accelerates the removal of necrotic tissue.

Granuflex is a hydrocolloid. When it comes into contact with wound exudate the hydrophilic particles swell and form an impermeable gel. This acts as a physical barrier and encourages the rehydration of necrotic skin. A change is evident within a few days, but total separation may take a few weeks, depending on the size of the area.

Debrisan is an alternative. This is a xerogel which absorbs excess exudate after contact with the wound. It produces a

Table 5.1 . Dressing types (this list is not exhaustive and dressings not listed may be in routine use in some departments)

Dressing type	Trade marks of some examples
Dry non-adherent	Melolin, N-A Dressing
Paraffin-impregnated gauze	Jelonet, Bactigras, Sofra-Tulle
Foam dressing	Silastic Foam, Lyofoam
Film dressing	Opsite, Tegaderm
Xerogel	Debrisan
Hydrogel	Geliperm, Intrasite Gel
Hydrocolloid	Granuflex
Alginate	Kaltostat, Sorbsan

moist environment without maceration of the wound. It does require a secondary dressing such as Opsite.

Infected wounds

The wound must be cleaned by irrigation with saline. The management will depend on the type and position of the wound and the capabilities of the patient. For minor infected wounds old-fashioned treatments such as regular salt bathing are effective and cheap! Difficult wounds may require more advanced dressings, such as Debrisan. Kaltostat is a calcium alginate dressing containing both the calcium and sodium salts of alginic acid prepared in fibre form. When moist the calcium alginate is converted to the soluble sodium salt, producing a hydrophilic gel. The dressing may be removed from the wound by simple irrigation or bathing in saline, and these dressings may therefore be more comfortable for the patient.

Sloughy wounds

There has been recent debate over the best agent to use on sloughy wounds. Hypochlorite solutions have been used for many years, but some authorities believe that they are ineffective and delay healing. In one of the few controlled clinical trials on the subject, the wounds treated with the hypochlorite healed as quickly as those treated with a modern wound dressing. Such solutions probably still have a place in the short-term (i.e. over a few days) cleaning of wounds.

Kaltostat, Intrasite Gel, and Granuflex are effective in cleaning sloughy wounds.

Granulating wounds

Dressings used on these wounds must provide a moist wound environment, and should not damage the tissue when removed. Paraffin tulle has been the traditional method for this type of wound care. However, care is needed to ensure that the dressing does not dry out, or else it may become very adherent. Opsite provides a moist environment, is impermeable to bacteria, and may be used on such wounds. Granuflex and Sorbsan are examples of newer dressings which may be used on granulation tissue.

Epithelializing wounds

Once the process of skin cover commences a moist atmosphere will encourage growth.

Paraffin tulle has been used with good effect, but the dressing must not be allowed to become dry, or it will adhere to the surface and on removal may pull off the fragile new epithelium.

Granuflex and Opsite and the foam dressings may also be of use on such wounds.

Problems with dressings

- **Skin sensitivity**
- **Interference with circulation**
- **Difficult removal**
- **Summary**

Skin sensitivity

Many of the more traditional skin adhesive dressings have a significant incidence of allergic reactions. Elastoplast is such an example. Always ask about skin sensitivity; if reddening develops after use, then use another method of securing the dressing, such as Micropore, a bandage, or Netelast.

The chlorhexidine in some medicated paraffin tulle dressings (e.g. Bactigras) may cause skin sensitivity.

Intrasite Gel contains propylene glycol, which may cause skin irritation.

Interference with circulation

Dressings and bandages may cause problems with venous return or even arterial supply if applied too tightly around a limb or digit. Take special care with crush injuries where swelling is inevitable and may cause a dressing to become too tight.

Try not to place non-stretch dressings or tape circumferentially around a finger.

Inform the patient to seek further medical advice if the dressing feels too tight or if severe pain occurs.

Difficult removal

The usual cause is that the dressing has become dry. This is made worse if there has been bleeding after application of the dressing, and dry blood clots may weld the dressing to the wound.

Good dressing technique, good haemostasis, and prevention of desiccation are the important steps to prevent such difficulties. In wounds where adherence may be a problem the polyurethane or silastic foams are less likely to adhere.

If a dressing does become adherent then soak in saline for 10 minutes.

The fingertip injury is one area where dressing adherence may make removal very difficult. One very good way of preventing this problem is the use of a flamazine finger-stall. Flamazine is put into the finger of a plastic glove and applied to the finger and secured. As with the flamazine hand bag (see Part 4 on burns management) the problem is that the wound and the surrounding skin become macerated. However, use of the dressing for a few days allows the wound to recover, and the initial dressing change is relatively painfree.

Other dressings, such as Kaltostat and Sorbsan, are said to be easier to remove.

Summary

There are many dressings available for the treatment of wounds. The routine dressing used in each department will vary, depending on the experience and personal preferences (or prejudices!) of the staff. Many of the newer dressings are expensive. Some of these may be cost-effective, however, since fewer dressing changes may be required.

References and further reading

1. Brown, J.S. (1997). *Minor surgery. A text and atlas*, (3rd edn). Chapman and Hall, London.

2. Bryant, R.A. (1992). *Acute and chronic wounds. Nursing management.* Mosby, St. Louis, MO.
3. Burge S., Colver, G., and Lester R. (1996). *Simple skin surgery* (2nd edn). Blackwell Science, London.
4. Flanagan, M. (1996). *Wound management.* Churchill Livingstone, Edinburgh.
5. McGregor, I.A. (1996). *Fundamental techniques of plastic surgery*, (9th edn). Churchill Livingstone, Edinburgh.
6. Spotnitz, W.D., Falstrom J.K., and Rodeheaver G.T. (1997). The role of sutures and fibrant sealant in wound healing. *Surgical Clinics of North America*, **77**, 651–68.
7. Thomas, S. (1990). *Wound management and dressings.* The Pharmaceutical Press, London.
8. Trott, A. (1991). *Wounds and lacerations. Emergency care and closure.* Mosby, St. Louis, MO.

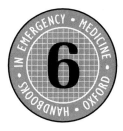

Wound infection

Prevention

Almost all wounds presenting to A&E departments occur in non-sterile conditions. The risk of wound infection is always present. Routine attention to the details of proper wound care minimizes the risk of wound infection. This involves:

1. Adequate history and examination to spot those wounds most at risk of wound infection, such as:
- wounds with delay to primary wound cleaning
- heavily contaminated wounds
- puncture wounds/bites
- wounds with tissue destruction

2. Alertness to constitutional factors predisposing to infection, such as diabetes, peripheral ischaemia, or immunosuppression.

3. Meticulous wound exploration and cleaning to remove contamination and necrotic tissue.

4. Careful closure to eliminate dead space.

5. Leave open heavily contaminated wounds with high risk of infection.

The organisms

The commonest organisms causing wound infection in A&E are *Staphylococcus aureus* and the beta-haemolytic streptococcus (*Streptococcus pyogenes*).

Staphylococcus aureus

Pathogenic staphylococci may be found in nasal swabs in up to 30 per cent of the population. The degree of virulence varies, but the typical lesion is one of local pus formation. The organism can enter the bloodstream giving rise to secondary pyogenic foci, septicaemic shock, or toxic shock.

Assume that the staphylococcus is resistant to penicillin. Most strains in A&E practice are still sensitive to flucloxacillin but the incidence of methicillin-resistant *Staph. aureus* (MRSA) is increasing in the community, especially in nursing homes. Other useful antibiotics in the treatment of staphylococcal infections are erythromycin (especially in the penicillin-allergic patients), cephalosporins, and clindamycin.

Streptococcus pyogenes

Although not so often isolated from wound swabs as the staphylococcus, this organism is probably responsible for many of the serious spreading infections seen in A&E. Spreading cellulitis and ascending lymphangitis often present primarily to A&E departments. Although many of these infections are easily treated, do not underestimate the virulence of this organism. It is the cause of necrotizing fasciitis and other invasive infections, such as pyogenic myositis, both of which can kill. Streptococcal infection can also cause potentially fatal septic shock and toxic shock.

It is very sensitive to penicillin. Erythromycin is the antibiotic of choice in those allergic to penicillin.

Mixed infections

Exposed wounds which are slow to heal may become colonized with the patient's own bacteria, usually resulting in a mixed growth of Gram-negative gut organisms.

Some wounds have specific infection risks. Human bites have a high incidence of anaerobic infection (*Bacteroides* group).

Prophylactic antibiotics

In normal A&E practice the routine use of antibiotics is NOT recommended in the management of uncomplicated wounds. There is no evidence that prophylactic antibiotics reduce the incidence of wound infection. Overuse will lead to resistance both within an individual patient and in the community as a whole. For example, *Staph. aureus* quickly became resistant to penicillin. It is still mostly sensitive to flucloxacillin, but the increasing resistance seen in hospital and in nursing homes would be disastrous if it became wide-spread in the community.

There are some definite indications for prophylactic antibiotics:

- open fractures (especially of fingertips)
- most mammal bites

Antibiotics are commonly given to patients with penetrating puncture wounds (e.g. 'stood on a nail'), but there is no evidence that this policy reduces infection risk.

Prophylactic antibiotics have previously been recommended for patients with valvular heart disease or prosthetic joints. It is no longer recommended that such patients receive prophylactic antibiotics for dental treatment and similarly they are not indicated in patients with simple uncomplicated wounds.

Relative indications are:

- wounds in agricultural workers or gardeners
- heavily contaminated wounds
- wounds with delay to treatment
- wounds with tissue necrosis

On logical grounds the best prophylaxis would be penicillin for beta-haemolytic streptococcus and flucloxacillin for *Staph. aureus*. However, oral penicillin is poorly absorbed, and in practice flucloxacillin is sufficient in the prophylaxis of both types of infection. A dose of 250 mg four times a day for five days is the standard course.

Erythromycin (250 mg four times a day) is the choice if the patient has a history of penicillin allergy.

In wounds where anaerobic bacteria may be a problem co-amoxiclav (Augmentin) has many advantages. It is also active against *Staph. aureus*.

Side-effects of antibiotics

Allergy As many as 1 in 10 people give a history of penicillin allergy. Although true anaphylactic reactions are rare, beta-lactam antibiotics should not be given to those with a history of penicillin allergy.

Diarrhoea This is a very common side-effect. It is usually mild, but can be severe and at times life-threatening (see below). The decision to continue antibiotic treatment in a patient with diarrhoea will depend on the clinical assessment, the severity of diarrhoea, and the risk of discontinuing therapy.

Pseudomembranous colitis Severe bloody diarrhoea in a patient taking antibiotics may be due to this condition, which can be life-threatening. It is caused by an overgrowth of *Clostridium difficile*, an organism producing a potent exotoxin. All broad-spectrum antibiotics can cause pseudomembranous colitis. Patients with severe diarrhoea should be admitted to hospital, especially if there is blood in the stool.

Jaundice This is reported with increasing frequency in patients taking ampicillin and co-amoxyclav. As many as 1 in 6000 patients may be affected. Jaundice occurs more frequently in patients being treated for more than 14 days, and patients over 65 years of age. While short courses of co-amoxyclav are still recommended for specific indications (e.g. dog bites), the risk of jaundice should be considered in any patient undergoing prolonged therapy.

Contraceptive pill There is a small risk that broad-spectrum antibiotics such as ampicillin might reduce the effectiveness of the oral contraceptive pill (OCP). Women using the OCP should be advised to use additional contraceptive precautions whilst taking the antibiotics and for 7 days after finishing the course.

Drug interactions—see Table 6.1.

Established wound infection

This may present in different ways: either

(1) the primary presentation may be with established infection, usually as a result of delay by the patient in treating the wound, or

(2) it may present as a complication of the treatment of the wound originally treated.

Table 6.1 . Drug interactions

Antibiotic	Drug	Effect
Erythromycin	Terfenidine	Cardiac arrhythmia
Erythromycin, metronidazole	Warfarin	Increased anticoagulation
Metronidazole	Alcohol	Vomiting
Erythromycin	Cimetidine	Deafness

Diagnosis. The cardinal symptom is *pain*. The pain of pus within the tissues is especially unpleasant.

Examination of a patient with suspected wound infection should include examination of:

- the wound and its surrounding area
- local lymph nodes
- temperature

> **IF A PATIENT PRESENTS WITH PAIN WHICH IS THROBBING IN NATURE AND KEEPING THEM AWAKE THEN ASSUME THAT PUS IS PRESENT UNTIL IT IS PROVEN OTHERWISE.**

The clinical findings will vary depending on the type of infection.

Local pyogenic abscess

There may be the typical changes of swelling, fluctuation, tenderness, and local erythema, all indicating pus within the wound.

Treatment. If the wound has been sutured then the sutures and all pus and dead tissue should be removed. Formal incision and drainage may be required. The wound should be thoroughly cleaned and irrigated, and an antiseptic dressing should be applied. The dressing should be changed daily until the wound is clean. The wound should then be allowed to heal by secondary intention. Antibiotics may be required in cases with:

- spreading cellulitis
- lymphangitis/lymphadenitis
- systemic upset
- patients in whom infection may be serious, such as diabetics, or patients with implants or valvular heart disease
- immunocompromised patients (including the HIV-positive)

Cellulitis

Spreading erythema, increased local temperature, and pitting oedema indicate spreading cellulitis.

Treatment. Open the wound to ensure no pus is present. Clean and irrigate the wound thoroughly, and apply an antiseptic dressing. Use a skin marker to draw the margins of the cellulitis.

If the cellulitis is not widespread and patients are not systemically unwell, they may be treated as out-patients. Give benzyl penicillin 1.2 g intramuscularly and a course of oral flucloxacillin (500 mg four times a day) or co-amoxyclav (375 mg three times a day) for 10 days. Another oral penicillin may be added to the above regimen if extra anti-streptococcal cover is thought necessary. If the patient is allergic to penicillin then use cefuroxime intramuscularly (there is a 10 per cent incidence of cross-sensitivity between cephalosporin and penicillin). Give erythromycin 500 mg four times a day.

Clindamycin is a very useful drug in soft-tissue infections, and is worth considering. It has gained a reputation for causing pseudomembranous colitis, but has been used successfully on a routine basis on large numbers of A&E patients, with a low incidence of side-effects. If the drug is used the patient should be kept under regular review to the end of treatment.

If there is any systemic upset then admit for intravenous antibiotics. Also admit patients with florid cellulitis.

If patients are allowed home they should be instructed to return immediately if the condition becomes worse, especially if they develop systemic symptoms. They must be reviewed by the A&E department or their general practitioners the following day.

Ascending lymphangitis

A 'red line' spreading proximally on a limb indicates lymphangitis. Enlarged local lymph nodes indicate lymphadenitis.

Treatment. In the early stages (erythema still distal to elbow/knee) out-patient treatment is possible. Use a similar regimen to that described on p. 98 under 'cellulitis'. If the 'red line' has spread proximally and if the axillary or groin lymph nodes are involved then admit the patient. If there are any systemic symptoms or significant pyrexia then admit the patient.

Again, if out-patient treatment is given the patient must be reviewed the following day.

Joint infection

The knee, hand, and finger joints are relatively superficial, and septic arthritis may be a sequel in penetrating wounds in these regions. If joint penetration is suspected then request X-rays looking for air within the joint.

Suspected septic arthritis is referred to the in-patient orthopaedic team.

Facial infections

Wound infections around the eye may lead to orbital cellulitis, with the potential complications of septicaemia or intracranial spread of the infection, including cavernous sinus thrombosis. Cellulitis complicating such wounds requires admission.

Systemic upset

Patients with systemic upset (a pyrexia above 38°C, 'shivering attacks' or flu-like symptoms) require admission for intravenous antibiotics and observation. Septic shock requires rigorous resuscitation and admission to intensive care.

Necrotizing fasciitis

This is a severe infection caused by some strains of *Streptococcus pyogenes*. The initial wound may be minor; even a grazed, bruised area can result in infection. The infection spreads rapidly through the subcutaneous tissues, deep fascia, or even within the muscles (pyomyositis), and may be well established within 12–24 hours. The early skin changes may be very subtle; slight erythema or mild induration may be the only signs. However, the patient is unwell, pyrexial, and complains of severe pain.

Patients with a history suggestive of necrotizing fasciitis should be referred to the in-patient plastic surgical team. These patients need immediate treatment with fluid replacement, high-dose intravenous penicillin, and immediate radical surgery to debride all the involved tissue. This may leave huge wounds, but such surgery is necessary as continued invasion will cause even more skin necrosis and may even kill the patient.

Toxic and septic shock

Some strains of *Staphylococcus aureus* and *Streptococcus pyogenes* produce potent toxins that can rapidly kill. Most cases of staphylococcal toxic shock have been associated with vaginal infection and tampon use. Streptococcal toxic shock occurs in small sporadic outbreaks due to the emergence of toxin producing sero-types. The entry wound may be minor, and in some cases there may be no apparent wound. The patient looks unwell, and will be pyrexial, with peripheral vasodilatation and hypotension. Treatment consists of surgical debridement, antibiotics, and intensive care.

Septic shock can result from any wound infection. The apparent ease of treatment of most wound infections should not allow doctors to become complacent and forget the virulence of these organisms which have the ability to kill fit, young individuals.

Tetanus

Tetanus kills large numbers of people each year in developing countries. (Estimates range from 50 000 to 2 000 000 deaths per annum.) Cases are rare in the UK, owing to the active immunization programme and good facilities for immediate wound care. However, cases do still occur (3 to 6 per annum), and meticulous attention to detail is required in the care of all wounds.

Clostridium tetani is an anaerobic Gram-positive bacillus. It lives in the gut of ruminant animals, and passes out into the soil in faeces. It forms spores, which are very resistant. The normal life cycle is that the ruminant ingests the spores, and multiplication takes place in the gut. The bacillus may be found in the human gut, where it acts as a commensal and does not cause disease.

The spores are ubiquitous, and it must be assumed that all wounds may be contaminated.

Tetanus is caused by the multiplication of the bacteria within a wound. The bacteria produce toxins, and it is the neurotoxin, tetanospasmin, which is responsible for the disease. The toxin diffuses up motor neurones to the central nervous system, where it blocks inhibitory control of the motor neurones. This results in tonic spasm of striated muscle. Other toxins, such as haemolysins, are also elaborated, giving rise to further tissue damage.

The mortality is highest at the extremes of life, with a shorter incubation time and increased severity of the disease. Death results from asphyxia or is due to cardiovascular collapse.

Prevention

Wound care The organism is anaerobic, and this underlines the importance of proper wound care. Dead tissue and haematoma are ideal culture media for the organism. Such conditions must be prevented by full wound toilet and good closure techniques.

Active immunization Tetanus can be prevented by inducing immunity to the tetanus toxin. Tetanus toxoid is a preparation of the toxin which has been inactivated and adsorbed on to aluminium phosphate or aluminium hydroxide. In the UK it is part of the routine immunization of infants. Therefore most people born after 1960 have been offered immunization, as have those who have been in the armed forces or those in certain occupations, such as miners.

Those who MAY NOT HAVE ADEQUATE IMMUNITY include:

- patients over the age of 40, especially women
- immigrants
- foreign nationals, especially those from developing countries
- patients with a history of vaccine refusal

ALL PATIENTS WITH WOUNDS MUST BE ASKED THEIR TETANUS IMMUNIZATION STATUS.

Warning Tetanus prophylaxis is important but often overlooked in burns, eye wounds, and when patients delay seeking treatment.

Immunization is not an 'all or nothing' response. The young and fit may mount a good response even 20 years after the last toxoid. However, the old and the immunocompromised may be unable to respond even when they have had a booster within 10 years.

The immunization schedule given in the following section is for the 'average case'. This may be modified given different wound factors or constitutional factors within the patient. Human immunodeficiency virus (HIV) will reduce the capacity to respond.

Allergy

Patients may say that they are 'allergic to tetanus injections'. This may be due to a true allergy, but the more likely explanation is that they have had a marked local response to a tetanus toxoid booster. These reactions can be very painful, with marked local pain, swelling, and local lymphadenopathy. They are more likely if the time interval between boosters is short. These reactions are usually self-limiting. Analgesics and systemic antihistamines may help.

The other 'allergy' may be found in older patients who may have been given horse tetanus immunoglobulin. Prior to the introduction of human immunoglobulin this was used to give passive immunity (see below). This practice has now been abandoned owing to the high incidence of allergic reactions.

There are few contraindications to tetanus toxoid. A completed course or booster within the past year is one contraindication. Pregnancy is NOT a contraindication. Do not give if the patient has an acute febrile illness unless they have a tetanus-prone wound. Peripheral neuropathy is a rare complication of tetanus immunization and there have been isolated reports of encephalopathy and transverse myelitis.

Passive immunity

If a patient has not received active immunization prior to wounding it will take some time before the toxoid will induce antibody production. There is a gap, therefore, in which clinical tetanus may occur.

Human tetanus immunoglobulin is harvested from blood donations, and is available as Humotet or from the Blood Transfusion Service.

If the patient is not adequately immunized and there is a high risk of tetanus then this can be given IN ADDITION to commencing active immunization.

Immunization

A course of tetanus toxoid consists of THREE injections (intramuscular) of 0.5 ml of tetanus toxoid at MONTHLY intervals.

A booster of tetanus toxoid is 0.5 ml of tetanus toxoid.
Tetanus immunoglobulin: the normal prophylactic dose is 250 units given intramuscularly at a different site to the toxoid. (This may be doubled if the risk of tetanus is severe or more than 24 hours have elapsed since injury.)

All babies are now offered tetanus immunization when 2 months old. This should be followed by boosters at 4 and 14 years of age. If this full 5-dose schedule has been completed then routine 10 yearly 'boosters' are **not** recommended.

Immunization on wounding

Table 6.2 sets out the recommended schedule for tetanus immunization in patients with a wound. The following wounds are regarded as TETANUS-PRONE:

- those where there has been a delay of more than 6 hours before adequate wound toilet
- those with evidence of sepsis
- puncture-type wounds
- wounds that have been in contact with soil or manure
- wounds with devitalized tissue

Treatment

Successful treatment of an established case of tetanus depends on speedy diagnosis. The early signs of the disease may not be impressive or specific. There may be no history of a wound in up to 30 per cent of cases. The incubation period is usually 6–10 days, but spores may lie dormant in the wound, to produce an infection some months after

Table 6.2 . Tetanus prophylaxis on wounding

Last booster/course	Clean wound	Tetanus-prone*
Less than 10 years ago	Nil	Nil/consider Immunoglob
More than 10 years ago	Toxoid	Toxoid + Immunoglob
Not immunized/unknown	Toxoid course	Toxoid + Immunoglob

* See above for definition of tetanus-prone wounds. Immunoglob: human tetanus immunoglobulin.
Penicillin may also be given for wounds at serious risk.

the injury. The specific symptoms which should alert the doctor to the possibility of tetanus are dysphagia and trismus (lockjaw). This is accompanied by fever, malaise, and headache.

Unfortunately this cluster of symptoms is not specific to tetanus. Severe mouth, throat, or jaw infections may give the same initial presentation.

As the disease progresses the more classical signs of rigidity of erector spinae, giving neck retraction and spasms of the facial muscles (risus sardonicus) develop.

Have a high index of suspicion in:

1. Those at high risk—agricultural workers, field sportsmen
2. Cases of deep wounds with tissue destruction
3. Non-immunized patients
4. Immunocompromised patients (from cancer, chemotherapy, or HIV)

Once the diagnosis is made the patient is admitted. Treatment consists of:

- complete exploration of the wound under general anaesthesia
- tetanus immunoglobulin in large doses (2000–4000 units)
- benzyl penicillin or metronidazole intravenously
- good supportive intensive care, with sedation to control muscle spasm and with assisted ventilation
- attention to fluid and electrolyte balance
- support of the myocardium if cardiac failure is present

Rabies

Rabies is caused by a rhabdovirus which travels to the brain via peripheral nerves. Although the disease is not endemic in the UK, cases do occur as a result of bites sustained abroad and one case of a rabid bat was reported on the south coast of England in 1996. Patients may also come to A&E departments for advice if they have been bitten abroad.

Rabies is endemic in all continents except Australasia and Antarctica.

The disease is mainly carried by carnivores, commonly dogs, foxes, and wolves. However, other mammals, including bats, may carry the disease.

Prevention

The disease may be prevented by immunization. There have been great improvements in rabies vaccine with the introduction of the human diploid cell preparation (HDCV).

Pre-exposure prophylaxis may be given to those especially at risk, such as vets and animal handlers who may come into contact with imported animals or may work in endemic areas. Information regarding this can be obtained from a consultant in bacteriology or infectious disease or from the nearest Public Health Laboratory.

Post-exposure prophylaxis may be indicated in patients returning from abroad and seeking advice in the A&E department. It may be possible to be certain that there is no risk of rabies from the history (animal known to be well one week after the bite, animal known to have been recently immunized). However, in the majority of cases there will be doubt, and in this situation POST-EXPOSURE PROPHYLAXIS MUST BE GIVEN, EVEN IF THE BITE IS A FEW MONTHS OLD. Seek the advice of a consultant in microbiology or infectious disease or of the Public Health Laboratory. If the patient has been bitten in a 'no-risk' country (see Table 6.3) then no immunization is needed. If bitten in a 'low-risk' area then 1 ml of HDCV is given and arrangements made for further follow-up. (If the patient is unimmunized they will require further doses on days 3, 7, 14, and 30.) Patients bitten in a 'high-risk' area will need HDCV and passive immunization with human rabies-specific immunoglobulin. (Advice may be obtained from the Virus Reference Laboratory, Central Public Health Laboratory, 0181 200 4400.)

Diagnosis and treatment

Diagnosis is difficult in the early stages unless there is a high index of suspicion. The incubation period lies between 20 and 90 days in 90 per cent of cases. The further the bite from the brain the longer the incubation.

Table 6.3 . Risk of rabies*

No risk	Low risk	High risk
UK, Ireland, Scandinavia, Spain, Portugal, Greece, Caribbean Islands, Japan, Singapore, Australia, New Zealand	France, Belgium, Germany, Switzerland, Netherlands, Denmark, USA, Canada	Mexico, South America, Africa, Asia

* For full information see *Immunisation against infectious disease.* Department of Health, 1996.

The initial symptoms are pain or paraesthesia at the site of a healed bite, along with fever, malaise, myalgia, and sore throat. The later symptoms are hydrophobia, inspiratory muscle spasm, and convulsions, although in some cases there is a flaccid paralysis.

Treatment. The mortality for established rabies is almost 100 per cent, although modern intensive care has led to a few successes.

Hepatitis B

Although this is not strictly an infection in a wound, it may be acquired through certain types of wound.

IT IS ESSENTIAL THAT ALL REASONABLE STEPS ARE TAKEN TO PREVENT EXPOSURE OF A&E PERSONNEL TO BLOOD DURING THE MANAGEMENT OF WOUNDS.
STAFF WORKING IN A&E DEPARTMENTS SHOULD BE OFFERED IMMUNIZATION AGAINST HEPATITIS B.

It is common to have health workers seeking advice regarding the risks of hepatitis B after accidental exposure to blood or other body fluids.

The risks are real. The virus may be transmitted by accidental inoculation (needlestick injury), by blood or saliva contamination of an open wound, or by a bite. Fortunately many health workers are now immunized against the virus.

A&E departments should have clear guidelines regarding the proper channels for the treatment of such cases. The first step is to follow the normal routines of wound care in terms of history, examination, cleaning, and tetanus immunization if indicated. Antibiotics will be required for human bites.

As with tetanus immunization, the treatment depends on the patient's immunization status and the risk of infection. Most hospital staff are now immunized and have a record of their response (a 'non-responder' will have anti-hepatitis B antibody titres of less than 10 mIU/ml). Previously immunized individuals may require a booster dose of hepatitis B vaccine following significant exposure. Unimmunized individuals require an accelerated course of hepatitis B (HB) vaccine and possibly hepatitis B immunoglobulin (HBIG), see Table 6.4.

An accelerated course of HB immunization consists of 3 doses, starting on the day of attendance, followed by doses at 1 month and 2 months (in contrast to the normal 3-dose schedule: day 0, 1 month, and 6 months). The injection is given intramuscularly in the deltoid area; the efficacy of the vaccine may be reduced if the buttock is used.

If HB immunoglobulin is given simultaneously with HB vaccine it must be administered at a different site.

Human immunodeficiency virus (HIV)

The risk of contracting HIV from a needlestick injury from a known HIV-positive source is 1 in 350. However, it is recommended that health care workers sustaining needlestick injuries from a HIV positive source (or strongly suspected to be HIV-positive) should be offered chemoprophylaxis. If this treatment is to be effective it must be

Table 6.4 • Post-exposure prophylaxis for significant exposure to blood or body fluids. (See text for details)*

HBV status of exposed person	Known HBsAg[1] positive source	Unknown source	HBsAg[1] negative source
Not immunized	HBIG Accelerated course HB vaccine	Accelerated course HB vaccine	Start course HB vaccine
Known responder to HB vaccine	Consider booster dose HB vaccine	Consider booster dose HB vaccine	Consider booster dose HB vaccine
Known non-responder to HB vaccine	HBIG Consider booster dose HB vaccine	HBIG Consider booster dose HB vaccine	Consider booster dose HB vaccine

* Adapted from *Immunisation against infectious disease.* Department of Health, 1996.
[1] Hepatitis B surface antigen.

given as quickly as possible after exposure, preferably within 1 to 2 hours.

A patient presenting with a needlestick injury from a HIV-positive source needs to be given a high triage priority; A&E departments should have guidelines about the counselling and treatment of these patients. If you are unsure then seek advice from A&E senior staff, or the departments of Occupational Health or Infectious Disease. The treatment consists of a combination of antiviral drugs, all of which have significant side-effects; thus it is essential that patients are adequately counselled about the risks and benefits before undertaking a course of treatment. The current recommendations for post-exposure prophylaxis are: zidovudine lamivudine, and indinavir.

Gas gangrene and synergistic gangrene

Gas gangrene

This infection is caused by anaeorbic bacteria of the clostridial group. These are often found in the guts of mammals, including humans, and in the soil.

The wounds most at risk are those with marked tissue destruction. War wounds are especially at risk, but the infection may be seen in severe crushing injuries or contaminated penetrating wounds.

The clostridiae produce a variety of exotoxins, haemolysins (lecithinase), collagenase, hyaluronidase, and deoxyribonuclease. These toxins cause local tissue necrosis and cellulitis. The muscles may putrefy. In addition the toxins cause shock, haemolytic anaemia, jaundice, and renal failure.

Clostridial septicaemia is a late and terminal event.

Prevention The lessons of prevention learned in the treatment of war wounds should be applied in the civilian situation where destructive contaminated wounds occur.

The wounds should be fully explored under general anaesthesia, all necrotic tissue should be removed, and the wound should be left open, to be closed only by secondary suture after it is clear that conditions are favourable. Prophylactic antibiotics are given (penicillin).

Treatment The diagnosis is made in a patient with a history of a severe wound in which there has been contamination and tissue destruction. The signs of local wound infection will be present. Gas may be felt in the tissues or may be seen on X-ray. The patient will be systemically ill, with signs of shock.

The patient should be vigorously resuscitated. High oxygen concentrations are given (hyperbaric oxygen is indicated, but it is unlikely that the ill patient will be fit to travel to one of the few units able to give this treatment). Large doses of benzyl penicillin are given.

Surgery must be carried out following resuscitation. Radical wound excision is performed. Amputation may be indicated in limb wounds. The wound is irrigated copiously with saline and left open. It is then inspected after 24 hours, and any further dead tissue is excised. This process is repeated until it is certain the infection is cleared, and only then may closure or skin grafting be carried out.

Synergistic gangrene

This is a serious infection caused by a mixed infection of aerobic and anaerobic or microaerophilic bacteria. The diagnosis is made by observing rapid spread of tissue necrosis and signs of toxaemia in the patient.

Commence 100 per cent oxygen therapy and broad-spectrum antibiotics. Urgent radical excision of the whole area is essential or life may be threatened. All affected skin is excised down to the deep fascia, until well-vascularized margins are obtained. Frequent reinspection is required, with excision of any further non-viable or suspect tissue. Only when it is clear that the infection has resolved should skin grafting be considered.

Non-healing wounds

If a wound is not healing despite reasonable treatment then a number of possibilities should be considered:

- The presence of *low-grade infection.*
- The presence of a *foreign body*—always take an X-ray if this is suspected. Wood, sutures, and plastic may not show on X-ray, and wound exploration may be required.
- *Underlying deep sepsis* such as osteomyelitis.
- *Poor vasculature*—either arterial or venous insufficiency may lead to long delays in wound healing, especially in the lower limbs. The risks of gangrene are increased. Great care is required in the treatment of wounds in such patients.
- *Steroid therapy*—delayed initial inflammatory response, reduced macrophage function, increased capillary fragility, and increased wound infection rates are some of the reasons which may delay healing in patients taking steroids. Such patients require careful observation.
- *Diabetes mellitus*—poor peripheral circulation, peripheral neuropathy, and interference with white blood cell function cause problems.
- *Dermatitis artefacta*—very occasionally a wound will fail to heal because of interference by the patient. Take care to exclude other reasons for non-healing listed above. A trial of plaster of Paris over the dressing may help confirm suspicions.

There are many rarer causes of non-healing wounds, such as neoplasia or pyoderma gangrenosa. If a wound is not responding to treatment ask for senior advice.

Further reading

1. Bisno, A.L. and Stevens, D.L. (1996). Streptococcal infections of skin and soft tissues. *New England Journal of Medicine*, **334**, 40–5.

2. Cummins, P. (1994). Antibiotics to prevent infection in patients with dog bite wounds: A meta-analysis of randomised trials. *Annals of Emergency Medicine*, **23**, 535–40.

3. Cummins, P. and Del Beccaro, M.A. (1995). Antibiotics to prevent infection of simple wounds: Meta-analysis of randomised studies. *American Journal of Emergency Medicine*, **13**, 396–400.

4. Department of Health (1996). *Immunisation against infectious disease.* HMSO, London.

5. Department of Health (1997). *Guidelines on post-exposure prophylaxis for health care workers occupationally exposed to HIV.* DoH, London.

6. Nicholson, K.G. (1997). Rabies. *Medicine*, **25**, 22–4.

7. Robson, M.C. (1997). Wound infection. *Surgical Clinics of North America*, **77**, 637–50.

8. Galazka, A. and Gasse, F. (1995). The present status of tetanus and tetanus vaccination. *Current Topics in Microbiology and Immunology*, **195**, 31–53.

PART 3
Management of specific wounds

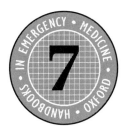

Special types of wounds

Puncture wounds

The commonest penetrating wounds in A&E practice are those of the limbs, especially the hands and feet. Sharp shards of glass, cutting tools, drills, and nails often cause such wounds. These deep, penetrating wounds may enter joints or tendon sheaths, and severe infections may result.

History. The exact nature of penetration is ascertained. A simple 'stood-on nail' is quite different from penetration by a high-speed metal fragment.

Examination. Often the wound is unimpressive, and there may be no direct evidence of damage to deep structures. Always look for signs of joint irritation (pain on passive movement) or tendon sheath involvement (pain on passive stretch or resisted movement).

Investigation. X-ray may be indicated, and is essential if a retained radiopaque foreign body or joint penetration is suspected.

Treatment. In deep puncture wounds the normal methods of wound toilet cannot be used. It is not advisable to perform extensive dissection to clean a puncture wound. The wound may be irrigated with saline using a needle to direct a jet of fluid into the wound. These wounds must always be regarded as contaminated, and have a high tetanus risk.

Full tetanus immunization is essential (see p. 104). Prophylactic antibiotics are often given although there is little evidence that they reduce the incidence of local infection. Ciprofloxicin may be the best antibiotic as many infections are due to *Pseudomonas* species.

Foreign bodies

The failure to diagnose a foreign body in a wound is a common reason for complaint and litigation.

Assessment

History will suggest if there is any possibility of retained glass/wood/metal.

If the wound was caused by glass establish if it shattered or if an unbroken edge incised the skin.

High-speed metal fragments may penetrate deeply, causing serious organ damage in eye and trunk wounds (see p. 19 and p. 176).

Identification of a wooden foreign body is difficult, since wood will not normally show on a radiograph. If patients consistently say they can feel a sensation of a foreign body within the wound then they are often correct. If in doubt ask for a senior opinion.

If a wound will not heal or suffers from persistent infections, then a retained foreign body should be suspected.

Careful *examination*, especially at the time of wound toilet, is mandatory.

Investigation: **X-ray is essential in all wounds caused by shattered glass, or crockery or metal fragments.** Wood will not be visible on X-ray unless covered with metallic paint. Ultrasound is advised when a radiolucent foreign body is suspected.

Treatment

If the foreign body is visible or easily palpable then it can usually be removed. If it cannot be seen or felt then seek further advice before exploring the wound. Although the foreign body may look easy to find on the X-ray it will take time and skill to locate. Most experienced doctors will agree with the saying 'the best person to remove a foreign body is someone else'.

If you do embark on such an exploration then ensure:

1. You have radiographs in two planes to show the position of the foreign body. These should be taken with two metallic markers forming a cross on the skin surface. The position of these markers should be marked on the skin with indelible skin marker. This allows accurate visualization of the relationship of the foreign body to the skin surface, and guides the placement of incisions (Fig. 7.1).
2. Adequate anaesthesia.
3. Bloodless field. It is very difficult to explore a continually bleeding wound.

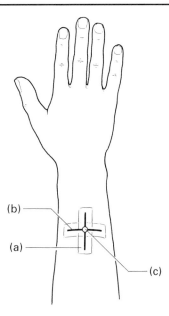

Fig. 7.1 . Surface marking for foreign body location, metallic markers. (a) and (b) are placed at right angles across the site of the pucture wound. (c) Enables accurate location of foreign body.

4. You have adequate instruments. Routine suture packs are inadequate. Fine instruments and some form of skin retractor are essential.

5. You have good light.

WARN the patient the foreign body MAY NOT be found. IF YOU ARE UNSURE THEN ASK SENIOR ADVICE.

Image intensifiers and ultrasound probes may assist foreign body localization, but are not routinely available in most A&E departments.

Bites

An average-sized A&E department will see between 400 and 500 animal bites per annum. Dog bites will account for over

90 per cent of mammal bites. The mouths of all animals are heavily colonized by bacteria, and all bites are therefore contaminated.

Dog bite

History. Some important points to note are:

1. The type of dog, and whether it was known to the patient. Large dogs with powerful jaws will inflict a greater degree of crushing and tearing of the tissues.
2. The time elapsed since the bite.
3. The tetanus immunization status of the patient.
4. Did the bite occur outside the British Isles?

BITES OCCURRING OUTSIDE THE BRITISH ISLES MUST BE IDENTIFIED, AND ADEQUATE RABIES IMMUNIZATION MUST BE GIVEN.

Examination. Perform routine examination and description of the wound. Damage to deep structures needs to be excluded. Large dogs may fracture bones, and joint penetration is possible.

Investigation. X-ray may be needed if bony injury or the presence of a foreign body such as a tooth is suspected.

Treatment

Wound toilet is performed. This may be difficult in puncture wounds. Copious saline lavage should be used.

Wound closure. It used to be standard teaching that dog bites should not be closed primarily. Many bites can be left open, and delayed primary closure may be appropriate. However, there are some bites which demand closure—for example, a gaping wound on the face. Such wounds may be closed, but they require meticulous wound cleaning, copious lavage, wound excision and careful technique.

Tetanus. Prophylaxis should be given as indicated.

Rabies. Immunization should be given if indicated.

Antibiotics. While many studies have shown no benefit from routine prophylactic antibiotics, a large meta-analysis has shown that they *do* reduce the rate of wound infection following dog bites. They must be given for:

- bites of hand
- if the wound has been closed primarily
- if the wound is penetrating
- if there is much tissue destruction

Co-amoxoclav (Augmentin) would be a suitable choice. If antibiotics are not given then the patient must be instructed to seek medical advice immediately if the wound shows signs of infection.

Human bites

These are potentially much more serious than dog bites. The human mouth is heavily contaminated with a mixed bacterial flora, including a number of anaerobic organisms. These wounds have a high risk of infection.

Treatment The wounds should be opened, irrigated, and left open. Beware of the small tooth wound over the metacarpophalangeal joints which results when a clenched fist meets an incisor tooth. Fifty per cent of these wounds will involve the metacarpo-phalangeal joint (see p. 146).

Prophylactic antibiotics must be given. These should cover both aerobic and anaerobic bacteria. Co-amoxoclav (Augmentin) would be a suitable choice.

It is essential to ensure the patient is adequately immunized against tetanus. Human bites may transmit the hepatitis B virus, though as yet there is no recorded case of transmission of HIV. However, if the person biting the patient is known to carry either of these viruses or has risk factors associated with the carrier state (institutionalized patients, male homosexuals, drug abusers) then seek further advice regarding management (see pp. 107, 108).

Cat bites

These have high potential for infection, and cat bites of the hand may give rise to joint or tendon sheath infections. *Pasteurella multocida* is the common infecting organism. It is very sensitive to penicillin.

Other mammal bites

The treatment consists of adequate wound toilet, lavage, and prophylactic antibiotics. Tetanus (and rabies) prophylaxis are given if indicated (see pp. 104, 106).

Insect bites

The common presentation is that of bites to the legs which blister and exhibit a marked local erythematous reaction. This is usually an allergic reaction, although it is difficult to be sure that there is not an infective component.

The local blister is aspirated, the wound is dressed, and an antihistamine is prescribed. If there is marked local cellulitis then an antibiotic may be added. The patient is instructed to elevate the leg.

Tick bites may transmit the organism causing Lyme disease (arthritis, skin rash, meningitis, and encephalitis). Patients with a history of tick bites should have prophylactic penicillin (erythromycin if allergic).

Wasp and bee stings may cause local swelling, but treatment is rarely required. The exception is the patient who may have severe allergic reactions to bee stings. This may present as anaphylactic shock.

- Give oxygen
- Give adrenaline (0.5 ml of 1 in 1000 solution by intramuscular injection)
- Give 200 mg hydrocortisone IV, and 10 mg chlorpheniramine IV
- Give IV fluid (e.g. 1 litre colloid stat)
- Admit the patient

Snake bites

The only indigenous venomous snake in the British Isles is the adder (*Vipera berus*). Its bites are seldom life-threatening. Sporadic exotic snake bites are seen with imported snakes.

First aid consists of attention to the airway, breathing, and circulation, and to the local treatment of the bite. The limb should be immobilized and kept elevated. Seek senior advice regarding the use of antivenom. (Advice may be obtained from Poisons Information Centres.)

The major effects of severe envenomation are vomiting, abdominal pain, diarrhoea, hypotension, and loss of consciousness.

Information on the bites of exotic snakes can be obtained from the London Poison Information Centre, or the Liverpool School of Tropical Medicine.

Flap wounds and pre-tibial lacerations
Problems

Wounds in the A&E department are not straight with well-defined edges. Flap lacerations present special problems. The blood supply of the flap may be compromised, especially if the base of the flap is more distal in the limb than the apex. The commonest example of this wound is the pre-tibial laceration in the elderly. The skin of this area is very thin and in a vulnerable area. Even minor trauma may turn back a large flap of thin skin.

Treatment of pre-tibial lacerations

There are many ways to treat such injuries EXCEPT by direct suture. This leads to delayed healing and increased complications. The standard treatment is to clean the wound, remove bruised and non-viable fat, and then use Steristrips to appose (NOT CLOSE) the wound. As in all flap lacerations, it is essential that the tissues are not placed under tension. Even using this method, part of the flap often dies. A Viscopaste® dressing is then applied and the patient instructed to rest and elevate the leg. The patient may be followed up in the A&E department or by the general practitioner, as appropriate.

Other methods include primary excision and grafting or defatting and meshing the flap, and reapplying as a graft to the defect. The decision to treat conservatively or by operative methods will depend upon the patient, the wound, and local facilities. Most of these wounds will heal with

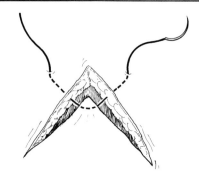

Fig. 7.2 . Suture apex flap laceration.

conservative treatment, but healing may take 2 to 3 months. Operative treatment will require admission to hospital and possibly a general anaesthetic, but it will allow the wound to heal more quickly.

Other types

The care of other flap lacerations will depend on the area involved and the quality of the skin. Almost all flap lacerations of the face should be sutured. Most flap lacerations in the young are sutured. Use few sutures with a special suture for the apex of the flap (Fig. 7.2).

Crush wounds

In such injuries the skin wound may appear relatively minor, but a significant crush injury often leads to more long-term problems than an incised wound. These injuries may cause skin necrosis, fractures, deep haematomas, muscle compartment syndromes and neuro-vascular injury (see Fig. 7.3).

Assessment

History. The important points are:

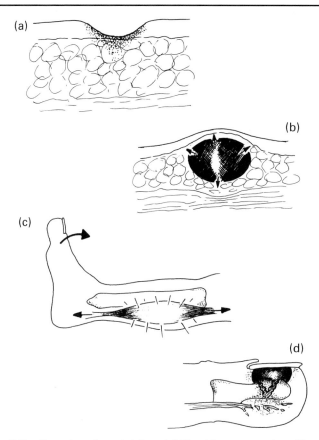

Fig. 7.3 • Sequelae of crush injury. (a) Direct trauma causing skin necrosis. (b) Pressure on skin from haematoma causing ischaemia and skin necrosis. (c) Pressure in fascial compartment causing muscle necrosis (compartment syndrome). (d) Crush fracture and trauma to nerve endings.

1. The exact mechanism of the crush. Visualization of the forces involved will give a good indication of likely tissue damage.

2 If the pain appears to be out of proportion to the physical findings then this may well indicate deep swelling and incipient compartment syndrome.

Examination. Pay special attention to the skin. Are there signs of skin ischaemia (white areas)? Are there signs of deep haematoma? Are there signs of degloving injury? Examine the movements of joints distal to the injury. Pain on passive movement of muscle groups under the wound may indicate compartment syndrome. Examine neurovascular function.

Investigation. X-rays are recommended in most significant crush injuries.

Treatment

After excluding fractures and deep damage, perform a careful wound toilet. These wounds may have significant amounts of dead tissue which require excision.

Wound closure. These wounds will swell. Use minimal numbers of sutures and do not tie too tightly. Some wounds may not close fully.

Aftercare. Patients are instructed on proper elevation techniques (p. 163) and to apply ice. They should return if the pain increases. Significant crush injuries should be admitted.

Skin necrosis The skin may die as a result of severe contusion, or due to a degloving injury which directly damages the blood supply. An underlying haematoma may cause skin ischaemia due to pressure effects. Skin necrosis often results from a combination of these mechanisms, and may take 3–14 days to become clinically obvious. Early signs include severe pain, poor capillary return, and a white appearance of the skin, especially in the middle of the wounded area. If large areas of necrosis are present the patient may require admission, and drainage of any haematoma (see below).

Subcutaneous haematomas If these are large and tense they may cause ischaemic necrosis of the overlying skin, leaving a large, deep defect which will take some months to heal. It is therefore essential to recognize this situation, and such haematomas should be incised, the haematoma evacuated, and a drain left in the wound. This often requires general anaesthesia. Needle aspiration is not effective.

Compartment syndrome This occurs when muscle swelling occurs beneath intact fascia. The leg is the commonest site, but it may occur in the forearm, the thigh, and even in the small muscles of the hands and feet.

THE sign of this injury is PAIN, especially on passive stretch of the affected muscle groups. If its presence is suspected then senior advice and admission is essential.

Open fractures

Classification

If there is a wound in association with an underlying fracture then it is best to treat it as an open fracture. Open fractures may be classified thus:

Grade I   Small skin wound, minimal soft tissue damage.
Grade II Moderate soft tissue injury, crushing force, comminution of bone.
Grade III Large wound, severe soft tissue injury, may have neurovascular damage.

Treatment

The most common open fracture is that of the terminal phalanx in crushing fingertip injuries. These are treated by thorough wound toilet, loose closure, and prophylactic antibiotics.

Other open fractures should be carefully assessed for distal neuro-vascular function. Gross deformity should be corrected, the wound should be cleaned by saline lavage and dressed with betadine soaks, and a splint should be applied. Intravenous antibiotics with high antistaphylococcal activity (e.g. cefuroxime) are given. Such major injuries will require admission for formal wound excision, cleaning, and fracture management.

High-pressure injection injuries

Pressurized paint, grease, or gas lines used in industry, or oil-based vaccines used in veterinary medicine may cause severe injuries. A patient presenting with a history of penetrating injury by such apparatus requires full assessment and referral.

The presenting wound may appear trivial, but the high pressure may have forced foreign matter for some distance up the limb following natural tissue planes. If these injuries are neglected then marked tissue destruction with loss of the limb is a possible sequel. These injuries will require extensive exploration of the limb to remove all traces of the material.

A detailed history and examination is followed by X-ray, tetanus immunization, and referral.

Needlestick injury

Increasing numbers of patients present with a history of needlestick injury. The patient's main concern is often about transmission of HIV or hepatitis B. Treat the wound as any other puncture wound, with thorough cleaning and tetanus immunization if required. Many departments have local guidelines on the management of needlestick injuries, but some general guidance is given below.

The risks of acquiring an infection from a community needlestick injury are very low, but an accelerated course of hepatitis B vaccine is recommended if the individual has not been previously immunized (see p. 108). HIV prophylaxis is not recommended for patients presenting with a community-acquired needlestick injury from an unknown source.

For details of hospital staff who sustain a needlestick injury see p. 108 (HIV) and p. 107 (hepatitis B).

Blood tests. If the source of the needlestick is known, consent may be sought for hepatitis B and HIV testing of the source individual's blood. This may aid the decision as to whether antiviral chemo-prophylaxis need be continued. A blood sample may also be taken from the injured patient for storage, but this is wholly for medico-legal reasons and will not affect the patient's immediate management.

Gunshot wounds

Characteristics of weapons

The damage to the body caused by a gunshot wound may be caused *directly* as the bullet passes through vital structures, or by the *transfer of energy* to the surrounding tissues.

The energy of a projectile is given by the formula: kinetic energy = $mv^2/2$; but there are other characteristics of the projectile, such as stability of flight, which will determine the amount of tissue damage.

The characteristics of common weapons are given below.

Airguns These are popular weapons, and cause the gunshot wounds most likely to be encountered in A&E departments. The pellets are small and the velocity low. Although visceral injury is possible, the pellets tend to pierce the skin and then follow tissue planes. There is not a great deal of surrounding tissue damage.

Handguns These use an explosive propulsive charge with subsequent higher velocity (150–250 m/s). The bullets are relatively large. They tend to penetrate viscera, causing direct damage along the path of the missile.

Shotguns Sporadic accidental injuries occur in rural areas, but injuries are more often the result of suicide attempts Shotguns are also being used increasingly in violent crime. They utilize an explosive propellant charge to fire a large number of small pellets. The extent of the injury is highly dependent on the distance of the target from the gun. At close range these weapons lead to devastating and often lethal wounds. As the range increases the damage decreases but the spread of the pellets may give wounds all over the body.

High-velocity rifles These weapons use small bullets but a very high velocity (up to 1000 m/s) to cause severe damage. The energy imparted sends shock waves through the tissues causing widespread tissue damage far removed from the path of the bullet. In the few milliseconds it takes the bullet to pass through the tissues a large amount of energy is transferred, resulting in a rapidly expanding 'temporary cavity'. Often clothing and other material is sucked into this wound. Tissues and organs distant from the track of the bullet sustain severe damage.

Management

Management is based on the care of the airway, breathing, and circulation. The principles are outlined under specific areas (see pp. 19–26). IMMEDIATE SURGICAL HELP IS NEEDED IN THE UNSTABLE PATIENT.

These wounds have a very high potential for tetanus infection, and adequate prophylaxis is essential. Antibiotics (parenteral penicillin) are given as soon as possible.

Airgun wounds may not cause significant damage. Peripheral airgun wounds may often be managed in the A&E department. However, if the wound involves the orbit, neck, chest, or abdomen further advice is recommended.

Most other gunshot wounds will require referral. Handgun injuries of the periphery may not require exploration if direct damage to vessels, nerves, or tendons can be excluded (this may require angiography). All high-velocity gunshot wounds will require extensive exploration that is outside the scope of the A&E department.

Records Such wounds are always the subject of rigorous police enquiry. Preserve all possible forensic evidence. All clothing is immediately placed in a bag clearly labelled with the patient's name and, if possible, with the name of the doctor or nurse who removed the clothing. Make full and accurate notes of all wounds or other injuries.

Blast wounds

Types of wounds

Explosions may cause complex injuries as a result of:

(1) direct penetration by fragments
(2) indirect blunt trauma caused by falling buildings or

caused by the victim being thrown some distance by the blast

(3) burns due to the heat of the explosion or a fire secondary to the explosion

(4) blast injury. This last is caused by high-pressure/ high-frequency sound waves. The energy in these waves is given up at the interface between media of differing density. In the patient this usually means between air in the lungs or bowel and the surrounding tissues

Management

A few 'explosions' such as the 'blow back' from domestic gas ovens can be easily managed, but the injuries caused by true explosions require senior assistance.

Management is based on stabilizing the patient by securing the airway, breathing, and circulation.

Burns of the face and airway may require immediate endotracheal intubation. Breathing may be hampered by direct chest injury such as pneumothorax or haemothorax, but the lungs may also suffer from the blast injury. The large number of air–fluid interfaces within the lung may produce a picture akin to a pulmonary contusion. High-flow oxygen is given, and endotracheal intubation may be required.

Shock is usually due to hypovolaemia, but exclude tension pneumothorax/cardiac tamponade. Secure venous access and commence fluid therapy.

Chest, neck, and pelvic X-rays are required. Check blood gases.

Perform a full head-to-toe survey describing all wounds. Pay specific attention to the chest (signs of blast injury may be slow in onset) and the abdomen (bowel blast injury).

If the patient is stable complete further investigations before transfer to the intensive care unit to allow close monitoring of lung function. The onset of lung blast injury will be noted by the detection of decreasing blood oxygen concentrations.

Further reading
Bites

1. Chadaev, A.P., Jukhtin, V.I., Butkevich, A.G., and Emkuzhev, V.M. (1996). Treatment of infected clenched fist human bite wounds in the area of the metacarpophalangeal joints. *Journal of Hand Surgery*, **21A**, 299–303.
2. Moore, F. (1997). 'I've just been bitten by a dog'. *British Medical Journal*, **314**, 88–9.
3. Steedman, D.J. (1994). Venomous bites and stings. In *Environmental medical emergencies*, pp. 189–99. Oxford University Press.
4. Wormser, G.P. (1996). Controversies in the use of antimicrobials for the prevention and treatment of Lyme disease. *Infection*, **24**, 178–81.
5. Ewan, P.W. (1997). Treatment of anaphylactic reactions. *Prescribers' Journal*, **37**, 125–32.
6. Cummings, P. (1994). Antibiotics and prevent infection in patients with dog bite wounds: meta-analysis of randomized trials. *Annals of Emergency Medicine*, **23**, 535–40.

Flap wounds

1. Haiart, D.C., Paul, A.B., Chalmers, R., and Griffiths, J.M.T. (1990). Pretibial lacerations: a comparison of primary excision and grafting with defatting the flap. *British Journal of Plastic Surgery*, **43**, 312–14.
2. Sutton, R. and Pritty, P. (1985). Use of sutures or adhesive tapes for the primary closure of pretibial lacerations. *British Medical Journal*, **290**, 1627.

Gunshot wounds and blast injuries

1. Paton, J.W.R. (1997). Ballistic injuries. In *Cambridge textbook of accident and emergency medicine* (ed. D. Skinner, A. Swain, R. Peyton, and C. Robertson), pp. 798–804. Cambridge University Press.
2. Hodgetts, T. *et al.* (1996). Blast and gunshot injuries. In *ABC of major trauma* (ed. D. Skinner, P. Driscoll, and R. Earlam) pp. 127–30. British Medical Journal Publications, London.

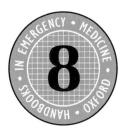

Hand wounds

Key points in hand wounds

Anatomy

Know it like the back (and front) of your hand.

History

How? When? Where?

Dominant hand? Occupation? Hobbies?

Glass and knives cut nerves and tendons.

Crush injury—? Fracture.

Foreign body still present?

Bites—high infection risk, especially for human bites.

High-pressure injury—always refer.

Examination

Describe wound.

NERVE INJURY IS FREQUENTLY MISSED—refer on index of suspicion.

Check tendon function, beware the 'boutonnière'.

Investigation

X-ray in glass and crush injury.

Treatment

Good light, good instruments, effective anaesthesia, safe tourniquet.

Splintage—'safe' position.

Always elevate.

Incised wounds

ENSURE NO NERVE/TENDON INJURY.

Primary closure in most cases.

Up to 1 cm diameter skin loss—dress. Larger area—seek advice.

Crush injury

Always 'worse than it looks'.

Exclude bony injury.

Minimal suture.

Elevate.

Fingertip crush

Children—treat conservatively.

Adults—may be treated conservatively.

If bone exposed will require skin cover.

Shearing

Severe injury—ask further opinion.

Nail injury

Drain subungual haematoma.

Replace 'levered out' nail.

Suture nail-bed laceration.

Tetanus

Always ask tetanus status and give appropriate cover.

Antibiotics

Always for bites.

Always for open fractures.

Follow-up

Advisable to follow up sutured wounds in the A&E department.

Hand injury accounts for 10 per cent of all A&E attendances—over one million new injuries per annum in England and Wales. The hand is a complex unit with vital sensory and motor functions, and these functions are often damaged by wounding. Residual symptoms and disability are common after seemingly 'trivial' hand wounds. Each wound must be fully assessed and treated appropriately.

The hand is capable of a vast range of activity, and each individual will place different demands on the hand. Consider other factors, such as the patient's occupation and hobbies, when deciding on treatment.

Anatomy

• **Surface anatomy**   • **Muscles and tendons**   • **Nerves**

There are few areas where a detailed knowledge of anatomy is as important as in the hand. Basic errors are often made because of lack of understanding of hand function, and doctors in A&E must have a sound knowledge of hand anatomy.

Descriptive terms NAME the fingers: thumb, index, middle, ring, and little. Numbering of fingers is *dangerous* and *not* acceptable.

Use the terms ULNAR and RADIAL to describe the borders of the wrist, hand, and fingers. The terms 'medial' and 'lateral' can be confusing (Fig. 8.1).

The palmar surface is referred to as the VOLAR surface and the back of the hand as the DORSUM.

Surface anatomy

The following figures show the relationship of some of the vital structures to the surface markings of the hand. Use these diagrams AND YOUR OWN HAND to identify these structures.

At the wrist many of the structures can be seen and palpated. Clench your fist and flex the wrist (Fig. 8.2).

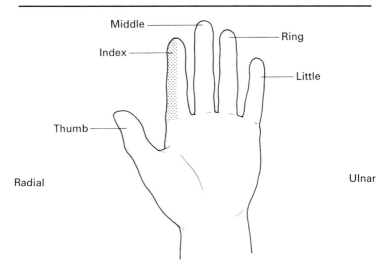

Fig. 8.1 • Naming of fingers and radial/ulnar aspects (shaded area = radial side index).

Flexor carpi radialis is the large tendon on the radial side of the wrist.

The *median nerve* lies on the ulnar (medial) side of the tendon and is superficial at this point, and thus easily damaged by penetrating injury.

The tendon of *flexor carpi ulnaris* can be seen (or becomes easier to feel) where it inserts into the pisiform bone (felt at the ulnar end of the distal wrist crease).

The *ulnar nerve* lies on the radial (lateral) side of this tendon. Press inwards on the radial side of the pisiform. This is uncomfortable, since you are pressing on the ulnar nerve.

Between the tendons of flexors carpi radialis and ulnaris lie the flexor tendon group. Flex and extend the fingers and these tendons will be seen moving.

The flexor tendons and the median nerve enter the carpal tunnel at the level of the distal wrist crease.

The skin of the palm is bound down to the deep fascia, and the tendons are hard to feel. The metacarpo-phalangeal

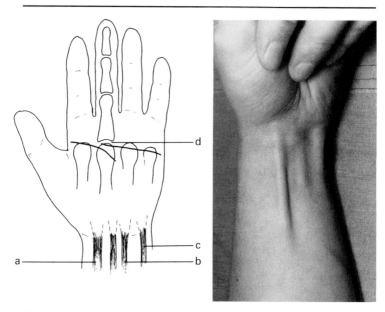

Fig. 8.2 • Surface anatomy at wrist. (a) Flexor carpi radialis. (b) Palmaris longus and finger flexors. (c) Flexor carpi ulnaris. (d) MCPJ at level of distal palmar crease.

joint (MCPJ) lies at the level of the *distal palmar* crease. At this level the finger bends into flexion, so this is an important point when placing splints or plasters to immobilize the hand. The flexor tendons may also be felt at this level. They are made more obvious by flexing the finger against resistance. This is an important landmark. The flexor tendon sheaths to the index, middle, and ring fingers commence at this level. The palmar digital nerves are just to each side of the tendon, and can be anaesthetized using these landmarks (see Figure 4.3, p. 51).

In the fingers there are three sets of flexion creases, at the level of the finger web (middle of the proximal phalanx) and over the proximal (PIPJ) and distal interphalangeal joints (DIPJ).

On the dorsum the skin is more lax and the structures more superficial. The radial and ulnar styloids are easily felt

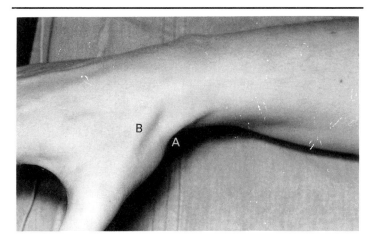

Fig. 8.3 . Structures on the radial side of wrist. (a) Extensor policis brevis/abductor policis longus. (b) Extensor policis longus.

at the wrist. (*Note* in turning the hand over that the radius now lies medial to the ulna: this shows the importance of using 'radial' and 'ulnar' rather than 'medial' and 'lateral' in describing injuries.)

The *anatomical snuffbox* lies distal to the radial styloid, bounded by the tendons of *extensor pollicis longus* (the obvious one on the dorsal/ulnar side) and the *extensor brevis and abductor longus* on the anterior aspect (Fig. 8.3).

Running over the radial styloid is the *radial nerve*, and the *radial artery* may be felt in the floor of the anatomical snuffbox. On the back of the hand the *extensor tendons* to the fingers are easily seen. The metacarpo-phalangeal joints are very superficial and easily penetrated.

On the ulnar border of the wrist the *dorsal (sensory) branch* of the ulnar nerve may be felt about one finger's breadth distal to the tip of the ulnar styloid.

Muscles and tendons

Fine control of finger movement is achieved by a delicate balance of muscular control by EXTRINSIC muscles (the long flexors and extensors with muscle bellies in the forearm) and the INTRINSIC muscles (muscles wholly within the hand, such as the interossei and the lumbricals).

Flexion of the MCPJ is by the INTRINSIC MUSCLES.
Extension of the IPJs is by the INTRINSIC MUSCLES (Fig. 8.4a).
Extension of the MCPJ is by the EXTRINSIC EXTENSORS.
Flexion of the IPJs is by EXTRINSIC FLEXORS (Fig. 8.4b).

Flexor tendons The extrinsic *flexor tendons* are flexor digitorum superficialis and flexor digitorum profundus. Over the middle of the proximal phalanx, superficialis tendon divides in two and inserts into the middle phalanx. The profundus tendon runs on to the distal phalanx (Fig. 8.5).

The deep flexor has one muscle belly, while the superficialis has separate bellies. Both tendons are important, profundus for power grip and superficialis for independent movement.

Extensor tendons The *extensor digitorum tendon* flattens to form the *extensor expansion*. It is joined at the level of the proximal phalanx by the tendons of the *lumbricals* and *interossei*. Over the PIPJ the expansion splits into three slips.

The *middle slip* inserts into the base of the middle phalanx, while the *outer slips* go on to the distal phalanx (Fig. 8.6).

The thumb has a slightly different arrangement. The *flexor pollicis longus* flexes the interphalangeal joint and the *flexor brevis* (intrinsic) flexes the MCPJ. *Extensor pollicis longus* extends the IPJ.

Nerves

The hand is supplied by the median and ulnar nerves, which have mixed motor and sensory functions, and the radial nerve, which is purely sensory in the hand.

The *median* nerve enters the palm on the radial side of the carpal tunnel. It gives the *motor branch* to the thenar eminence and then splits into the *digital* nerves, which supply the volar digital nerves to the thumb, the index and middle

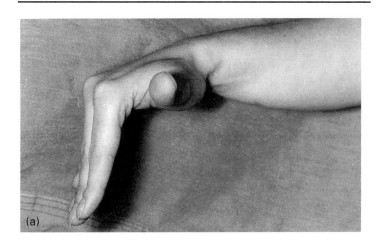

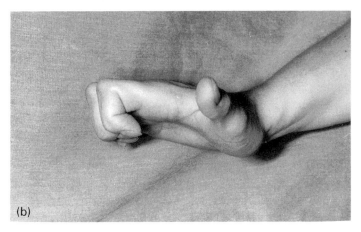

Fig. 8.4 . (a) Actions of intrinsic muscles of the hand. (b) Actions of extrinsic muscles of the hand.

fingers, and the radial part of the ring finger. It also supplies the radial two lumbricals.

The *ulnar nerve* enters the palm on the radial aspect of the pisiform bone. Above the wrist it gives off the *dorsal sensory branch*, which supplies the ulnar part of the dorsum of the hand and the dorsal digital nerves to the little finger and

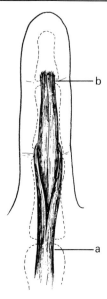

Fig. 8.5 • Anatomy of flexor tendon. (a) Flexor digitorum superficialis dividing. (b) Flexor digitorum profundus insertion to distal phalanx.

half of the ring finger. The ulnar nerve supplies ALL THE INTRINSIC MUSCLES OF THE HAND except those of the thenar eminence and two lumbricals. It therefore supplies all the interossei, two lumbricals, the hypothenar muscles, and adductor pollicis.

The *radial nerve enters* the hand over the radial styloid and gives the dorsal digital nerves to the thumb, the index and middle fingers, and half of the ring finger.

Table 8.1 • Summary of prime movers of joints

Joint	Flexion	Extension
MCPJ	Intrinsics	Extensor digitorum
PIPJ	Flex. superficialis	Intrinsics (middle slip)
DIPJ	Flex. profundus	Intrinsics
Thumb IPJ	Flex. pollicis longus	Extensor pollicis longus

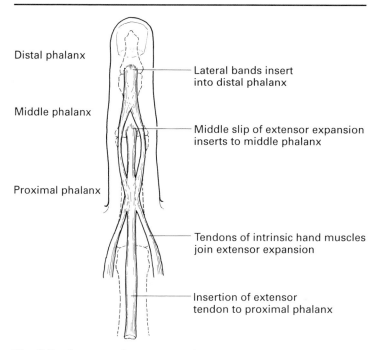

Distal phalanx

Lateral bands insert
into distal phalanx

Middle phalanx

Middle slip of extensor expansion
inserts to middle phalanx

Proximal phalanx

Tendons of intrinsic hand muscles
join extensor expansion

Insertion of extensor
tendon to proximal phalanx

Fig. 8.6 • Anatomy of extensor tendons.

Table 8.2 • Summary of nerve distribution in the hand (may vary)

Median	*Sensory* to volar surface of thumb, index, and middle fingers
	Motor to thenar eminence (opponens, short abductor)
Ulnar	*Sensory* to little finger and ulnar half of ring finger
	Motor to other intrinsic hand muscles
Radial	*Sensory* to dorsum of thumb, index, middle, and ulnar half of ring fingers

Assessment

- History • Examination • Tendon injury
- Flexor tendon injury
- Extensor tendon injury
- Nerve injury • Investigations

History

Proper management is not possible without a detailed history of the mechanism of injury.

The *how*? *when*? and *where*? are asked. There are certain points in the history which may have a major bearing on management.

Ask which is the patient's *dominant hand*. An injury to a dominant hand will usually cause more disability than injury to the non-dominant side. However, there are some occupations which require both hands; the left little finger of a guitarist is of vital importance. The occupation, hobbies, and pastimes of a patient may well alter treatment decisions.

Glass and knives cut. Assume damage to deep structures until it is proved otherwise.

Crush injuries may not produce large wounds but they cause a lot of tissue damage and swelling. There may be associated fractures. Such injuries often cause more longterm disability than incised wounds.

Foreign bodies are common in hand injury. Thorns and wooden splinters may be especially difficult, since they are often not visible on X-ray. If the patient is adamant they can feel something in their finger always take this seriously and seek further advice. Such foreign bodies often give rise to serious infection.

Bites of the hand may give rise to serious infection. Of special importance is the injury caused by punching someone in the teeth! There is often a small inconspicuous wound over the dorsum of the MCPJ, caused as the clenched fist strikes the incisor teeth. Such injuries often go through the extensor tendon and penetrate the joint. Septic arthritis and a finger amputation are possible outcomes if this injury is not managed correctly.

Pneumatic tools and *high-pressure grease guns* may only cause a tiny wound in the skin. Injection of grease, oil, veterinary vaccines, or paint under high pressure causes widespread tissue damage, and such a history will call for specialist referral.

Examination

Proper examination and description of the wound must be performed. It is essential to state which hand is injured and to NAME fingers. It may be possible to examine the full depth of the wound at this point. However, bleeding or haematoma may prevent full wound inspection, which must then be carried out during wound cleaning. Do not forget this important examination (see p. 157). If the task of wound closure is delegated then it is *your* responsibility to ensure that adequate wound inspection is carried out.

The testing for damage to deep structures is of special importance in hand injuries. Both partial and complete divisions of major nerves and tendons are often missed. This leads to a poor result and increased disability for the patient. With all hand wounds, but especially with incised wounds, assume damage to deep structures.

Always thoroughly inspect hand wounds.

Tendon injury

- **Flexors profundus and superficialis**
- **Flexor pollicis longus** • **Extensor digitorum**
- **'Boutonnière' deformity** • **Mallet finger**
- **Extensor pollicis longus**

Flexor tendon injury

Damage to the long flexor tendons may be evident from just looking at the resting hand. Examine your own hand at rest. The fingers are slightly flexed at all three joints. Division of both flexor tendons will result in one finger's sticking out straight. Each flexor tendon should be tested in turn.

Profundus tendon is easiest to examine. Lie the patient's hand on a flat surface and hold the finger straight by gentle pressure on the middle phalanx area. Using the other hand ask the patient to flex the DIPJ against the resistance of

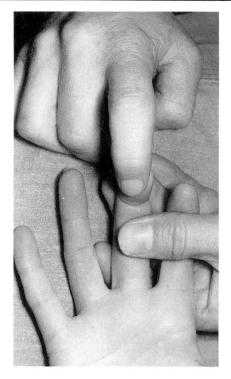

Fig. 8.7 . Testing flexor profundus. Resisted flexion of the DIPJ.

another of your fingers (Fig. 8.7). Inability to do this indicates division. Pain on resisted flexion may indicate PARTIAL DIVISION OF THE TENDON.

Flexor superficialis is more difficult to test. The profundus tendon will also flex the PIPJ, and must be 'disabled' to allow testing of the superficialis function. This is done in the following manner:

Assume the middle finger is to be tested.

- The hand is placed flat and palm upwards.
- The index, ring, and little fingers are held extended.
- The MCPJ of the middle finger is also held extended

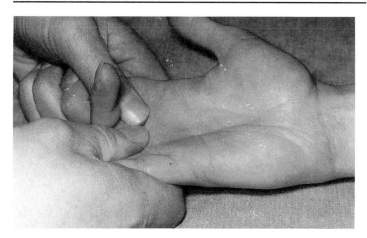

Fig. 8.8 . Testing flexor superficialis.

(remember flexion at this joint is due to the intrinsic muscles).

- The patient is asked to flex the finger, and the finger should flex only at the PIPJ.
- The DIPJ will be 'floppy' since flexor profundus, having a single muscle belly, is inactivated by holding the fingers straight (Fig. 8.8).

This test may not always be reliable with the index finger, since some people have a separate profundus belly to the index finger.

The tendons to each finger are tested in turn.

Flexor pollicis longus is tested by flexing the IPJ of the thumb against resistance.

Extensor tendon injury

Division of *extensor digitorum* is detected by the inability to extend the MCPJ (Fig. 8.9a). (Remember that the PIPJ and the DIPJ can still be extended through the action of the intrinsic muscles.)

Damage to the central slip of the extensor tendon over the PIPJ is difficult to diagnose. Wounds (or blunt trauma) in this

(a)

(b)

(c)

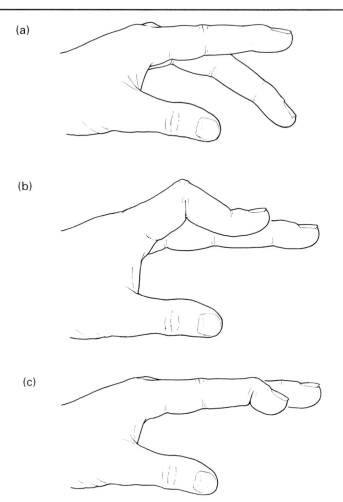

Fig. 8.9 • (a) Metacarpo-phalangeal joint extensor lag in the middle finger due to division of the extensor digitorum tendon to that finger. (b) Boutonnière deformity of the index finger due to division of middle slip of extensor expansion. **This deformity may appear some weeks after injury**. (c) Mallet finger due to division/rupture of extensor tendon to distal phalanx.

region may divide the central slip. At initial presentation extension may appear NORMAL because of intact lateral bands. Specific tests of central slip function are notoriously unreliable. With the MCPJ slightly flexed, downward pressure on the dorsum of the proximal phalanx will produce extension of the digit if the central slip is intact. However, a careful history and high index of suspicion remain the mainstay of diagnosis at this stage. If a cut is present over the dorsum of the PIPJ it should be examined very carefully for evidence of damage to the extensor tendon.

If the diagnosis is missed, the lateral bands displace to the side of the joint over the following weeks, and begin to act as flexors. The result is the boutonnière deformity (Fig. 8.9b). Once established, this deformity is exceedingly difficult to treat.

The *extensor expansion* can also be damaged over the DIPJ. Such damage is easy to diagnose, owing to the loss of extension at this joint ('mallet finger'—Figure 8.9c).

Extensor pollicis longus is tested by extension of the IPJ and by feeling the intact tendon as it crosses the anatomical snuffbox.

Nerve injury

> • **Sensory testing** • **Motor testing** • **The radial nerve**

It would seem impossible that division of an important structure such as the median nerve might be overlooked. However, such nerve injuries are only too easy to miss. The signs of nerve injury may take some time to become obvious. There is evidence that action potentials may still cross the cut nerve for up to 24 hours. Moreover, the patient may not be able to believe that he cannot feel part of the hand. An accurate history will indicate those wounds with a high likelihood of nerve injury (glass and knife wounds), and this finding should be followed by meticulous examination.

Sensory testing The sensory fields of the three nerves are summarized in Figure 8.10.

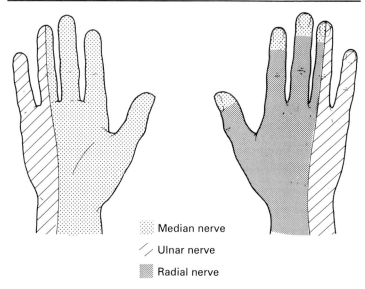

Median nerve
Ulnar nerve
Radial nerve

Fig. 8.10 . Sensory distribution of nerves to hand.

Test the sensation in the NORMAL hand. Using the normal hand will ensure that the patient understands the test and can co-operate.

- Ask the patient to close his or her eyes (to remove the possibility of visual prompting interfering with the examination).
- Test three sensory modalities: light touch (cotton wool), pin prick (special disposable needles are recommended), and two-point discrimination. Compare with the equivalent area on the uninjured hand.
- The test should then be repeated on the injured hand.

> **NOTE: SENSATION MAY ONLY BE SLIGHTLY ALTERED, and such a finding is significant if found in the expected anatomical distribution.**

Sweating will also be absent if a nerve is cut. This may be felt directly by the examiner's finger, but may also be noted by lightly drawing a pen top down the tip of the finger and comparing the sensation with that felt when doing the same to a normal finger. The lack of sweating will alter the 'feel' of the resistance of the skin.

Tests such as electrical skin resistance are not routinely available in A&E departments.

Motor testing *Motor function—ulnar nerve*: test finger adduction.

Place the hand flat on a surface and ask the patient to hold a piece of paper by adducting the fingers. If the ulnar nerve is divided then the paper can easily be removed (Fig. 8.11a).

A further test is that of thumb adduction (Froment's test). The patient is asked to grip a piece of card between the thumb and the base of the index finger. If the adductor pollicis is not functioning then the IPJ will flex as the patient uses the flexor pollicis longus to perform the movement (Fig. 8.11b).

Testing abduction of the index finger is also a good indicator of ulnar nerve function (Fig. 8.11c).

Motor function—median nerve: test opposition and abduction of the thumb.

Asking the patient to touch the tip of the index finger with the thumb, observe the plane of the thumbnail during this movement. During rest the thumbnail is at right angles to the plane of the palm. As opposition takes place the thumb rotates so that the nail lies parallel to the palm (try it on your own hand) (Fig. 8.12a).

Thumb abduction is tested by asking the patient to press up and against a pen held parallel to the palm of the hand. The muscles of the thenar eminence are palpated during abduction, and the short abductor should be felt to tighten (Fig. 8.12b).

The radial nerve This is often damaged in wounds over the radial styloid. Although division of this nerve is not important functionally, damage may lead to troublesome neuroma

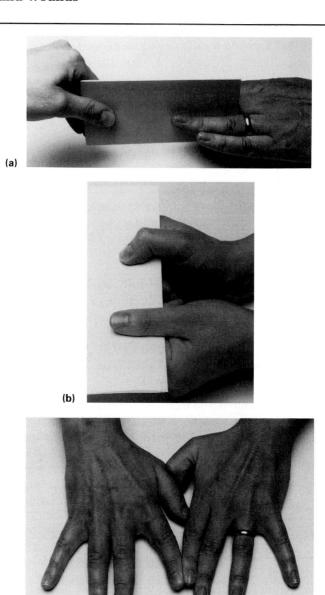

(a)

(b)

(c)

Fig. 8.11 • Testing ulnar nerve function. (a) Finger adduction. (b) Froment's test. (c) Index finger abduction.

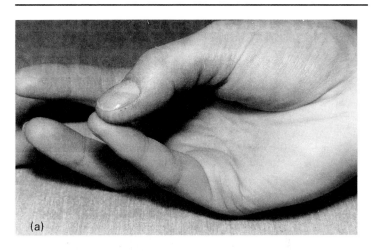

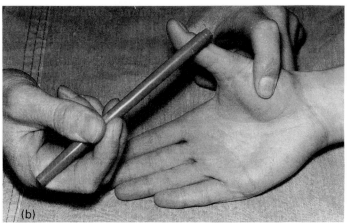

Fig. 8.12 . (a) Thumb opposition. (b) Testing short abductor of thumb.

formation. Injury is diagnosed by testing sensation over the dorsum of the first web space.

All the steps listed above require time, patience, and a co-operative patient. There are real difficulties in the assessment of such injuries in young children, in those with learning difficulties, and in the drunk. If in doubt ask for further advice.

Investigations

The commonest investigation will be radiography. It is indicated if there is possibility of a radiopaque foreign body such as glass or metal. Wood will not normally appear on a radiograph (unless it has traces of metallic paint). Crush injuries should be X-rayed to exclude fractures.

Treatment: general principles

- **When to refer** • **Instruments** • **Anaesthesia**
- **Wound examination** • **Tourniquets**
- **Dressings and splintage** • **Elevation**

When to refer

Most hand injuries are treated in the A&E department. However, before deciding to treat a wound take into account all the factors referred to above, such as the site of injury, dominance, occupation, age, and hobbies.

If damage to *deep structures* is suspected then this *should be referred for a further opinion.* A&E departments will vary in the type of hand injuries which they manage. Some departments have experienced hand surgeons, access to theatre and magnification equipment, and experienced physiotherapy departments to aid with rehabilitation. Even in such departments senior help and advice are recommended at an early stage. However, in most A&E departments tendon and nerve injuries will be referred to surgeons with a special interest in hand injury.

Instruments

A&E departments use small general-purpose suturing packs for most injuries. Such instruments may be satisfactory for a minority of hand wounds, but if delicate or complex work is required it is highly advisable that appropriate instruments are used. Packs should be available which contain finer forceps, fine dissecting scissors, skin hooks, and small retractors.

A comfortable patient and good light are essential. Assistance will make the task much easier, but is often in short supply in a busy A&E department.

Anaesthesia

Good anaesthesia is needed for adequate wound inspection, cleaning, and closure. Normal infiltration techniques may be used over the wrist and palm, but in the fingers there is little space to inject even small volumes of local anaesthetic.

Therefore, some form of nerve block is required. The most commonly used is the *metacarpal head block* (see p. 50). Whatever technique is used it is *VITAL* that PLAIN ANAESTHETIC SOLUTIONS ARE USED. **NO** adrenaline should be used in the hand. Adrenaline-containing solutions should be kept separately from other local anaesthetic solutions to prevent inadvertant use and possible loss of fingers.

Details of finger blocks are given in Chapter 4 (pp. 49–51).

Wound examination

Failure to carry out proper wound examination is the usual reason why injuries are missed. Care must be taken to achieve adequate local anaesthesia, good light, and a bloodless field; in addition, appropriate instruments are essential. Although these standards may be difficult to achieve, they are essential in order to provide proper wound care. When examining the wound consider the mechanism of injury. What was the position of the hand when it received the injury? Put a finger through its full range of movement; this may reveal tendon damage which would otherwise go unnoticed (Fig. 8.13).

Tourniquets

Good surgical results require good conditions. Wounds in the hand bleed profusely, and this makes accurate wound inspection and repair difficult. A watchmaker would not be asked to repair a watch at the bottom of a full inkwell! The ideal conditions for hand surgery are a fully exsanguinated

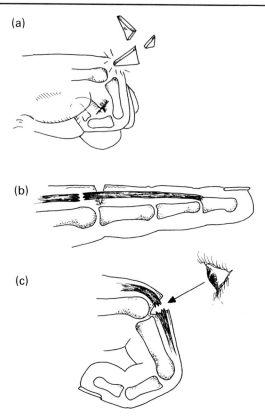

(a)

(b)

(c)

Fig. 8.13 . (a) Position of hand at time of injury. (b) Examination with finger extended. Tendon damage concealed proximally. (c) Flexion of the finger reveals tendon damage.

limb, regional anaesthesia, and an upper-arm tourniquet. Such conditions are mandatory for all serious hand injuries.

Most finger wounds and some hand wounds may be treated using local blocks and a finger or upper-arm tourniquet.

Great care and attention to detail are required during the use of tourniquets. Times of application and removal must be noted. Patients have left hospitals with finger tourniquets still in place. Keep tourniquet time down to a minimum.

The safest finger tourniquet is to use a *surgeon's glove*. The

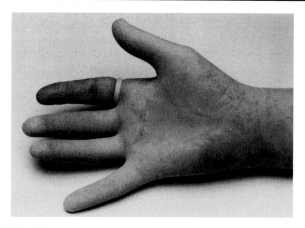

Fig. 8.14 . Finger tourniquet using a sterile surgeon's glove.

tip of the glove is cut off and then the glove is rolled down the finger to the base (Fig. 8.14).

Rubber catheters have been used for many years, but the pressures developed under these catheters can be excessive, and they are best avoided.

The use of an upper-arm tourniquet with a local hand block is possible for short periods. It is uncomfortable for the patient, but 15 to 20 minutes of operating time are possible in most patients. The technique is not suitable for young children.

Organization and routine are the key to successful use of the technique.

1. Explain the procedure to the patient.
2. Give local anaesthetic as described above.
3. Wrap the site of application of the tourniquet with cotton padding.
4. Apply the pneumatic tourniquet and check the inflation pressure needed to obliterate the radial pulse. (But note that the safe maximum of 50 mmHg above the patient's systolic blood pressure should not be exceeded.)
5. DEFLATE the tourniquet.

6. Elevate the arm while the operator washes, prepares the instruments, and ensures that everything is ready for the procedure.
7. With the arm still elevated wash and prepare the wound.
8. The tourniquet is then inflated and the operative procedure commenced. NOTE THE TIME.

See Figure 8.15 for a summary of this procedure.

This approach will not allow long periods of application of the tourniquet, but does provide good conditions for the repair of minor injury or foreign-body removal (but see the section on foreign bodies, Chapter 7 pp. 119–121).

Dressings and splintage

The main problem with hand dressings is that they will cause immobility and joint stiffness. Indeed, if the hand is immobilized in the wrong position for more than two weeks crippling joint contractures may develop.

If it is necessary to immobilize the hand injury then care should be taken to place the hand in the 'Edinburgh position'. The MCPJs are flexed and the IPJs are fully extended. The method of applying such a dressing is shown in Figure 8.16.

Elevation

There is no doubt that a high-arm sling makes the patient look as though he or she has sustained a serious injury. Equally, there is little doubt that a sling is a very POOR method of effective elevation. The hand is little higher than the heart and, more importantly, the elbow is bent, restricting venous outflow.

Swelling occurs in all hand wounds, but is especially damaging in crushing injuries. The patient must be instructed to elevate the limb in a proper fashion (Fig. 8.17). The arm is best rested on some pillows on the arm of a chair. This will achieve height, good venous return, and comfort.

The pain caused by swelling is extremely unpleasant and difficult to control by analgesia. Proper elevation and the

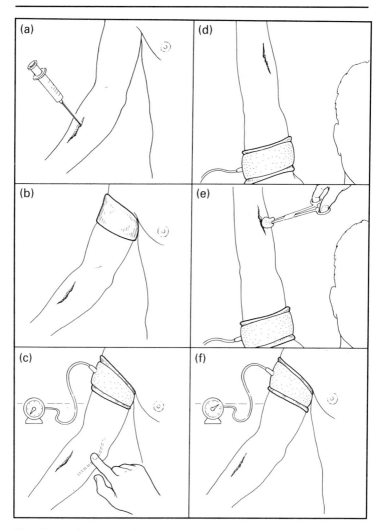

Fig. 8.15 • Summary of tourniquet procedure.

prevention of swelling will certainly lead to a happier patient, and probably also to a quicker recovery.

If the crush injury has been severe then the patient may require hospital admission for full elevation.

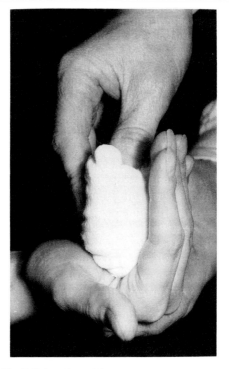

Fig. 8.16 . The Edinburgh position.

Treatment: specific wounds

- Incised wounds: no skin loss
- Incised wounds: skin loss
- Crush wounds: no tissue loss
- Crush wounds: tissue loss • Trapdoor flaps
- Amputations • Shearing wounds
- Nail injuries • Infected wounds

Incised wounds: no skin loss

Exclude nerve and tendon damage.

The wounds should be thoroughly cleaned, inspected, irrigated, and closed if possible.

(a)

(b)

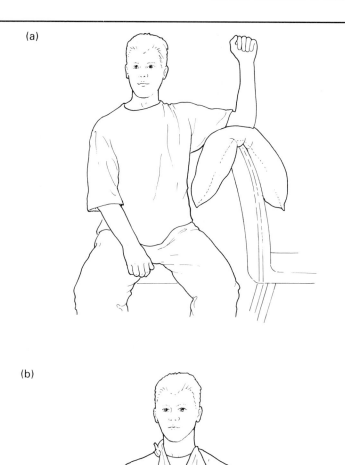

Fig. 8.17 . Arm elevation. (a) Proper position for reduction of hand swelling. (b) Poor position for reduction of hand swelling.

Inspection is often difficult because of bleeding. Tourniquet use is very helpful. The wound should NOT be extended unnecessarily. Wounds, especially those on the volar surface, may cause severe functional problems as a result of wound contracture. The unplanned extension of a wound by a doctor not trained in hand surgery should not take place in the A&E department.

Clean thoroughly. Do not excise hand skin unless it is completely non-viable. There is little 'spare skin' in the hand. All particulate matter should be removed.

Closure. Uncomplicated incised wounds are usually treated easily by simple suture. Accurate apposition of the skin edges is important. Do not tie sutures too tightly. Hand injuries give rise to significant swelling, so allow for this during closure.

Exclude tendon/nerve damage.

Incised wounds: skin loss

Such injuries occur on the fingertips and are often caused by knives or meat-slicing machines. Normally, the area of loss is small (less than 1 cm in diameter), and there is no bone exposed. The majority of these injuries can be treated conservatively. After wound toilet the area is dressed with a moist non-stick dressing. This is left undisturbed for 7–10 days. Although healing may be prolonged, the skin is of better quality than that of a skin graft.

If there is a flap which is only loosely attached, remove the fat from the undersurface of the flap and place the flap back in position. It may take as a free graft; if not, it provides an ideal dressing for the raw area and will separate as healing progresses.

Larger areas of skin loss and cases where there is exposed bone will require more definitive surgery, such as V–Y plasty or skin grafting. These procedures are not suitable for routine use by inexperienced junior A&E staff, and senior opinion is advisable.

Crush wounds: no tissue loss

Assume a crush injury is more severe than it appears. There is often little or no swelling and surprisingly good function when the hand is seen soon after the injury. However, these injuries often cause more long-term symptoms and disability than does a more impressive large incised wound.

A crushing force will not only damage skin, but also the highly specialized subcutaneous structures: fine nerve-endings, vessels, and bone.

The wounds in such injuries will have been produced by 'bursting' or by shearing of the tisues.

In the burst-type wound the wound must be thoroughly cleaned. Protruding fat may be removed with sharp scissors. Obviously dead skin should be removed; do not excise large amounts of skin. If possible these wounds should not be sutured. Adhesive skin strips (applied LONGITUDINALLY if possible) are extremely useful in realigning tissues. If sutures are necessary, then keep them to a minimum and tie them loosely. Finally the wound is dressed and instructions are given on proper techniques for elevation.

Crush wounds: tissue loss

The commonest injury is that to the fingertip as a result of crushing in a door or a machine.

In *children* the best method of treatment is by the conservative method. The wound is cleaned and dressed. The fingertip will regrow. Not only will this obviate the need for operation, it will give a normal finger as a result.

In *adults* the decision is more difficult. The conservative treatment of minor amputations is an option, but due consideration must be given to the configuration of the wound and other factors, such as occupation/hobbies. If *bone is exposed* then it is advisable to perform some procedure to provide soft tissue cover over the bone end. A scar adherent to bone is exceedingly tender, and produces very significant disability. In addition, maintaining length often improves the function of the digit, and primary closure will get a manual worker back to work more quickly than elaborate techniques. If in doubt seek further advice.

Trapdoor flaps

These result from with tangential slicing injuries through the skin, usually on the palm. Such injuries often heal with uneven skin edges, with one skin edge proud in relation to the other. Try to ensure the skin edges are brought level during suturing; if in doubt ask senior advice.

Amputations

Distal amputations are treated as described above. More serious amputations will definitely require referral. Often the amputated finger is brought to the hospital. Ensure this is correctly handled by placing it in a plastic bag which is then placed in water and ice (do NOT place the finger directly into ice).

Shearing wounds

These may be severe injuries, since the skin may be degloved. One example is that caused by a ring's being pulled up a finger. The skin may be completely degloved, and sometimes the finger must be amputated.

Such severe injuries will require senior opinions and inpatient treatment.

Nail injuries

Crushing injuries may produce an acutely painful *subungual haematoma*. The nail is exquisitely tender. This is easily treated by trephining the nail.

The best method is to use a number 11 scalpel and rotate this in a boring fashion. This creates a large-diameter hole. The alternative is to use the same spinning/boring method with a wide-gauge hypodermic needle.

More severe crushing may result in a damage to the nail-plate. The nail may be levered out of the nail-fold. Exclude fracture of the terminal phalanx. The nail should be replaced beneath the fold.

If the nail-bed has been severely lacerated it may require suture. This will require very good operating conditions, with adequate anaesthesia, a tourniquet, and fine instruments. In children this will often require a general anaesthetic. Great care is used in removing the nail. Use sharp-pointed scissors and gently separate the nail from the bed, pointing the scissors up into the nail avoiding further damage to the nail-bed. Wash the nail in saline.

Repair the laceration with fine 6/0 absorbable suture and then REPLACE the NAIL. The nail acts as a splint, prevents adhesions forming in the nail-fold, and is an excellent dressing for this extremely tender area.

Infected wounds

Special care is required in suspected hand infections. Figure 8.18 summarizes the infections which commonly occur after certain wounds. The classical sign of fluctuation is often NOT present. THE signs of hand sepsis are the typical throbbing pain and exquisite local tenderness. If not diagnosed these infections may give rise to serious local tissue damage, and they may lead to septicaemia.

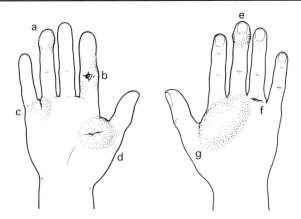

Fig. 8.18 • Infection of the hand following wounds. (a) Finger pulp space infection following wound to tip of finger or beneath the nail. (b) Tendon sheath infection following penetrating wound to volar aspect of the finger. (c) Web space infection following wound to base of finger. (d) Thenar space infection following wound to thumb. (e) Acute paronychia. (f) Incisor tooth wound to metacarpo-phalangeal joint resulting in septic arthritis. (g) Generalized swelling of dorsum of hand, found in most serious wound infections.

The signs of flexor tendon sheath infection are:

- finger is held in a flexed position
- tenderness over the tendon
- extreme pain on passive extension of the finger

Have a high index of suspicion, and always advise exploration of such wounds. Paronychia and pulp space infections may be incised under digital nerve block; but for more proximal infections formal exploration under general anaesthesia is required.

Further reading

1. Evans, D.M. (1989). The management of skin injuries of the hand. In *The practice of hand surgery* (ed. D.W. Lamb, G. Hooper, and K. Kuczynski), pp. 121–49. Blackwell Scientific Publications, Oxford.
2. Helal, B. (1989). Injuries to the finger tip. In *The practice of hand surgery* (ed. D.W. Lamb, G. Hooper, and K. Kuczynski), pp. 291–7. Blackwell Scientific Publications, Oxford.
3. Lamb, D.W. (1989). General principles of the management of hand injuries. In *The practice of hand surgery* (ed. D.W. Lamb, G. Hooper, and K. Kuczynski), pp. 111–20. Blackwell Scientific Publications, Oxford.
4. Anderson, I.W.R. and Sen, A. (1997). Hand injury. In *Cambridge textbook of accident and emergency medicine* (ed. D. Skinner, A. Swain, R. Peyton, and C. Robertson), pp. 589–600. Cambridge University Press.
5. American Society for Surgery of the Hand (1990). *The hand: Examination and diagnosis.* Churchill Livingstone, New York.
6. Chang, P. (1997). Nail bed repair. In *Techniques in hand surgery* (ed. W.F. Blair), pp. 82–7. Williams & Wilkins, Baltimore, MA.

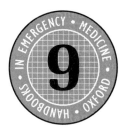

Facial wounds

Key points in facial wounds

1 Secure the airway early in severe facial wounds.
2 Exclude damage to deep structures:
   • Full neurological examination.
   • Skull and facial bone X-ray where appropriate.
   • Examine neck and X-ray where clinical signs indicate.
   • Full eye examination.
   • Check facial nerve function.
   • Examine parotid duct.
3 Treatment:
   • Most wounds can be managed in A&E, but care is needed.
   • Meticulous wound cleaning, with all dirt removed.
   • Layered closure of muscle and skin gives best results.
4 Specific wounds needing care:
   • Scalp wounds—exclude fracture/brain injury.
   • Eyelid wounds—refer if they cross the lid margin.
   • Eye wounds—meticulous eye examination.
   • Lip wounds—align vermilion border.
   • Nose wounds—exclude septal haematoma.
   • Ear wounds—beware bleeding from the ear, and refer pinna haematoma.

Introduction

Facial wounds are often alarming to the patient. The rich blood supply of the face means that these wounds bleed freely, with dramatic results. However, the correct application of basic wound management often leads to gratifying results, and the repair of most facial wounds will be possible within the A&E department.

Severe facial wounds due to blunt trauma are unusual in modern A&E practice. The compulsory use of seat-belts for the front-seat occupants of cars has lead to a dramatic reduction of 'windscreen face', where severe lacerations and fractures were often seen. The seat-belt legislation is one outstanding example of preventative medicine brought about, in part, by A&E specialists.

Resuscitation

Airway

Severe blunt facial trauma with compromise of the airway is one of the most challenging emergencies encountered. The patient is hypoxic and thrashing around, with blood everywhere, and with an abnormal airway anatomy.

Call for help immediately. Senior A&E staff and a senior anaesthetist must be involved at the earliest opportunity with such patients.

Initial management. If the patient's other injuries allow, log-roll the patient into a stable lateral position (NOT the formal recovery position). Tilt the trolley head-down.

Use suction to remove blood from the upper airway. If the mandible is fractured the airway should be maintained by the chin-lift manoeuvre rather than the jaw thrust.

High-flow oxygen is given.

Such simple manoeuvres will often improve the situation to allow adequate preparation for endotracheal intubation. This should be performed by the most experienced person available, and another doctor should be ready to perform cricothyroidotomy if oral intubation fails.

Once the airway is secure then proceed to the assessment of the breathing and circulation. Facial wounds bleed profusely, but simple external pressure will stop this. Life-threatening bleeding may occur in fractures of the middle third of the face, as a result of laceration of the maxillary artery. This can be identified by a severe nasal haemorrhage which will not stop with packing or balloon tamponade. These patients must be seen immediately by a senior ENT or facio-maxillary surgeon.

Assessment

History

The history of the wound is of paramount importance. Not only may blunt injury damage the facial skeleton and teeth, but transmitted forces may cause brain injury and spinal injury.

Ask if there has been any period of loss of consciousness or other symptoms such as nausea, vomiting, or diplopia.

Cutting injuries may well damage deep structures; glass wounds, especially from a shattered windscreen, should be assumed to have a foreign body within them.

Examination

The size and depth of wounds are noted. The deep structures of the face whose function must be tested are the facial nerve, the parotid duct, the lacrimal duct, and the eye. Beware of wounds in the extended triangle shown in Figure 9.1. Remember to look inside the mouth. Teeth may be broken or fractured. This examination will also alert you to the possibility of jaw fractures.

Carry out a full neurological examination, including recording of the Glasgow Coma Score (see Table 9.1). In severe injury ensure the neck is properly examined.

The branches of the facial nerve are outlined in Figure 9.1. Penetrating injuries and glass and knife wounds in the region of the facial nerve call for accurate assessment of the function of the facial muscles. Any suspicion of facial

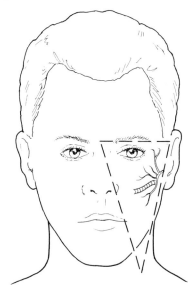

Fig. 9.1 . 'Triangle of danger' for facial wounds. The branches of the facial nerve, parotid duct, lacrimal apparatus, and contents of the orbit are at risk from injury.

Table 9.1 . Glasgow Coma Score

Eye opening		Verbal response		Best motor response	
Spontaneous	4	fully orientated	5	obeys commands	6
To voice	3	confused	4	purposeful movement to pain	5
To pain	2	inappropriate words	3	withdraws from pain	4
No response	1	incomprehensible sounds	2	flexes to pain	3
		no response	1	extends to pain	2
				no response	1

nerve injury requires consultation with the plastic surgery team.

The parotid duct lies in the middle third of the line joining the external auditory meatus and the angle of the mouth. If there is a deep cut in this region, suspect parotid duct injury.

Examine the parotid duct orifice from within the mouth (opposite the second upper molar tooth). If there is blood in the orifice damage is confirmed and immediate referral is required.

Investigations

Skull radiography may be required for scalp wounds. The absolute indications are:

(1) a history of loss of consciousness
(2) a diminished conscious level
(3) if the galea is breached or a fracture is palpable
(4) if there are neurological signs
(5) if there is a leakage of cerebrospinal fluid from ear or nose

Relative indications are: significant scalp bruising or swelling; and a history of a heavy object falling on the head (as, for example, in a building site injury).

If glass has caused the wounds then soft tissue tangential radiographs are requested.

Facial views. If damage to the facial skeleton is suspected request specific 'facial views' to show fractures of the maxilla, or specific mandibular views.

General principles of treatment

Meticulous wound toilet is absolutely essential in facial wounds. If dirt is left in the wounds then permanent tattooing will result. Severe grazes may need to be scrubbed, and if the area is large then general anaesthesia may be required. Damaged or contused wound edges should be debrided. Failure to do so may result in poor quality scars, slower wound healing, and an increased risk of wound infection. When debriding facial wounds great care must be taken to conserve as much tissue as possible.

Most significant facial wounds will require suture. Some minor wounds, especially in children, may be glued, but this technique is only suitable for small, superficial wounds which come together without undue tension (for details of technique see p. 77).

If the wound is deep then a carefully placed deep layer of sutures is used to repair the facial muscles and to bring the wound together, so that a line of small sutures is all that is required to appose the skin edges. If the deep layer is correctly placed then skin sutures may not be needed, and adhesive skin closures may be used.

Semi-circular wounds have a tendency to produce a 'trapdoor' scar with swelling of the encircled tissues. If closure as a linear wound can be achieved then this should be attempted. If you are unsure, ask for help from a senior colleague or refer to the plastic or facio-maxillary surgeons.

Scalp wounds

Scalp wounds may indicate damage to the skull or brain, and therefore a careful history and examination the required (see above). Be especially careful in wounds caused by heavy objects falling from a height—a brick, for example. This may cause an open depressed skull fracture, but the patient may walk into the A&E department. It is easy to underestimate the severity of such wounds.

The other major problem with scalp wounds is bleeding. This may be so severe that intravenous replacement may be required.

Bleeding is controlled by direct pressure. If the wound is large and deep and bleeding is severe, then a number of artery forceps may be applied to the galea, and this structure may be turned over the wound edges.

Deep wounds will require a layered closure, or a deep haematoma will develop.

Eye wounds

Assessment

The assessment of eye wounds requires strict adherence to routine if sight-threatening wounds are to be properly managed.

History *Intraocular foreign body.* Ask specifically if there is any history of hammering/using a chisel or other circumstances which may indicate a penetrating foreign body. Small penetrating wounds of the globe may give little immediate pain or disability, but complications may lead to the loss of the eye; in some cases the other eye may develop a sympathetic ophthalmitis, leading to complete loss of vision. Always take a history of possible penetrating injury seriously.

If the patient has felt something go into the eye while hammering, using a chisel or engaged in an activity where high velocity fragments are likely then ASSUME THE PATIENT HAS AN INTRAOCULAR FOREIGN BODY.

Tetanus prophylaxis is often overlooked in eye injury; always ask if the patient is adequately immunized.

Histories of *allergy* and *other illnesses* and *medications* are taken. It would be negligent to dilate the pupil for examination in a patient with a history of acute glaucoma.

Examination *Visual acuity.* The examination of a wound of a finger would be regarded as totally inadequate if the function of the finger was not tested.

IF THE VISUAL ACUITY IS NOT TESTED THEN A PROPER EXAMINATION OF THE EYE HAS NOT BEEN PERFORMED.

When the eyelids are swollen, it is important to test visual acuity and inspect the cornea and anterior chamber at the earliest possible stage, before the swelling closes the eye completely. If the patient presents with the eye completely closed, it is usually possible to carefully open the eye sufficient to allow examination. If this proves impossible, it is vital to arrange for a proper examination to be carried out as soon as the swelling subsides.

When patients present without their glasses, a pin-hole may be used to remove refractive error. Ask for a senior opinion if you have difficulty assessing a young child, especially if you suspect a significant eye injury.

General examination. Examine the eye, noting the colour of the conjunctiva, the clarity of the cornea, and the shape and reactions of the pupil. Blood may be seen in the anterior chamber (hyphaema). Examine the whole extent of the conjunctiva. The upper lid must be everted.

Fluorescein. Wounds of the conjunctiva and cornea will be more obvious if a vital dye is used to stain the epithelial defect. Instil fluorescein drops followed by normal saline (ENSURE CONTACT LENSES HAVE BEEN REMOVED). Wounds and corneal epithelial damage will fluoresce when examined with a cobalt-blue light.

Other examination. Examine the ocular movements, papillary reactions to light, and accommodation. Test visual fields by confrontation.

Examine the fundus, but remember that the whole of the fundus cannot be examined in most A&E departments. Even by dilating the pupil using cyclopentolate or another short acting cycloplegic the periphery of the fundus cannot be seen. It is in this region that traumatic retinal detachment will occur. Cases of significant blunt trauma should be referred to the ophthalmology department for indirect fundoscopy.

Investigations. The most important investigation is the plain radiograph, which MUST be taken if there is a suspicion of a retained intraocular foreign body.

Treatment

Patients with significant eye injury should be reviewed by the ophthalmologists. The list below indicates the conditions which require immediate referral:

- Eyelid wounds crossing the lid margin
- Wounds over the inner canthus (lacrimal duct)
- All penetrating wounds of the globe
- Deep corneal lacerations
- Alkali burns of the cornea

- Blood in the anterior chamber (hyphaema)
- Pupil irregularity/loss of pupil reflexes
- Vitreous haemorrhage
- Retinal detachment (hard to diagnose—refer significant blunt trauma to exclude this)

However, most wounds around the eye may be successfully treated in the A&E department.

Lid lacerations

A wound which crosses the lid margin, those through both surfaces of the lid, and those which may have damaged the lacrimal gland or duct should be referred (see Figure 9.2).

Most eyelid lacerations can be sutured without difficulty. Appose the edges accurately. Do not tie the sutures too tightly. Cut the ends of the suture shorter than normal, or leave them long and tape them out of the way, to prevent corneal abrasion.

Wounds of the eyebrow present few problems and are closed by suturing or glue. DO NOT shave the eyebrow.

Foreign bodies

If the upper lid is not everted then it is easy to miss a foreign body, and this procedure must be performed if the patient complains of something in the eye.

Most conjunctival foreign bodies are easily removed. Corneal foreign bodies are more difficult. They are often embedded in the epithelium. The cornea is only 0.5 mm

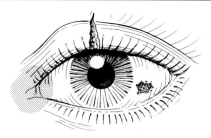

Fig. 9.2 • Eyelid laceration across lid margin. **Refer for senior advice.**

thick in some areas. The use of a slit lamp is extremely helpful. Some form of magnification is recommended. Amethocaine is instilled into the conjunctiva. Superficial foreign bodies may be removed by a moist cotton bud. A hypodermic needle mounted on a 2-ml syringe is the best method to remove an embedded foreign body, but its use requires great care and a co-operative patient. If the foreign body is not easily removed then the use of a slit lamp is essential.

After removal use fluorescein to check for corneal damage, and prescribe a topical antibiotic.

Metallic foreign bodies may leave a 'rust ring' of staining on the cornea. These are easier to remove after 2–3 days, and may be referred to the ophthalmic department.

Corneal abrasions

These will heal as long as infection is prevented. Ensure that deeper structures have not been damaged. Prescribe a topical antibiotic. If painful pupillary spasm is present then dilate the pupil using homatropine. If the vision is reduced then review is recommended.

Chemical burns

Patients with chemical burns to the eyes should be immediately triaged for urgent, copious lavage. Apply a topical anaesthetic and run at least one litre of sterile saline over the conjunctiva. Refer immediately if the cornea is not clear or if there are areas of blanching of the normal vascular pattern around the limbus (where the sclera meets the cornea).

Nose wounds

Blunt injury

Nasal injuries are often the result of blunt violence, most often by a fist. The common injury is that of nasal fracture, with or without an external laceration. Examination will determine patency of the airway, any deviation of the septum or nasal bones, and complications such as a septal haematoma.

Septal haematoma (easily seen as a red bulge emerging from the septum, blocking both passages) should be referred urgently to the ENT team for formal drainage.

Nasal fractures or septal injury should be referred to the ENT, plastic or facio-maxillary surgery out-patient clinic between 5 and 10 days.

Lacerations are sutured, and prophylactic antibiotics are given if a fracture is present.

Severe blunt trauma may cause more severe fractures of the facial skeleton, which may involve the cribriform plate, resulting in cerebrospinal fluid rhinorrhoea. If this is suspected then obtain X-rays of the facial bones and refer.

Full-thickness lacerations involving the alae (sides) of the nose require careful suture and, if severe, referral to the plastic surgery team.

The essential step in suturing these wounds is to appose the junction of the skin and mucosa very accurately. Any malalignment will be very obvious when the wound has healed. The first suture should be placed at the margin, and then the mucosa, cartilage, and skin should be sutured in layers.

Lip and mouth wounds
Lip

Most external lip wounds will require suture. If the wound is deep then the orbicularis oris muscle may be involved, and this should be repaired. If the wound crosses the junction of the lip and facial skin (vermilion border) then it is ESSENTIAL that this is accurately aligned if a noticeable 'step' in the lip margin is to be avoided. Always begin suture of such wounds by placing a suture to achieve this (Fig. 9.3)

Beware 'through and through' wounds. Both the deep layers and the external wounds must be repaired. The mucosal layer may be sutured or left to heal spontaneously.

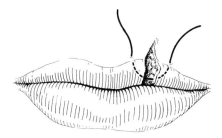

Fig. 9.3 • Suturing of lip laceration. Place the first suture accurately to oppose the vermilion border.

Teeth

If a lip is cut then careful examination of the teeth is needed. If a tooth has been knocked out then it must be found. It may be lost on the ground, but it may also be in the lip wound or have been inhaled into a bronchus. If the tooth is lost then a chest X-ray or a soft-tissue X-ray of the lip may be required.

If a patient brings a tooth which has been recently knocked out then it should be rinsed in warm saline and replaced into the socket. Urgent dental referral is essential.

If the tooth is fractured or loose then dental referral is advised to ensure adequate splintage.

Tongue

Minor wounds of the tongue do not require suture. Large tongue wounds are difficult, and senior opinion or referral is advised.

Ear wounds

Cartilage wounds

Most wounds of the pinna can be sutured in the A&E department. Wounds involving the cartilage, however, require special care. Infection in the cartilage leads to perichondritis, with destruction and ugly deformity. Meticulous wound toilet is therefore essential, and antibiotic cover is recommended.

Bleeding from the ear

Bleeding from within the ear should be fully assessed. The common traumatic causes are:

(1) a wound of the auditory canal from an instrument pushed into the ear
(2) injury to surrounding structures, such as a forceful dislocation of the temporo-mandibular joint
(3) perforation of the ear-drum
(4) a fracture of the base of the skull

A good history and examination will help identify the cause. Perforation of the ear-drum is often found after a slap over the ear. Such tears will heal spontaneously, and no treatment is required.

Fracture of the base of the skull will follow significant trauma, and will require careful assessment to exclude intracranial complications.

Haematoma

Although not strictly a wound, a haematoma of the pinna (boxer's ear) deserves special mention. The bleeding may separate the cartilage of the ear from the perichondrium. Attempts at aspiration always fail. The correct treatment is to refer these to the ENT or plastic surgeons. A small window is cut in the cartilage, and a small suction drain is placed to evacuate the haematoma.

Further reading

1. Hawksford, J. and Banks, J.G. (1994). *Maxillofacial and dental emergencies*. Oxford University Press.
2. Cooling, R.J. (1997). Ocular trauma and emergencies. In *Cambridge textbook of accident and emergency medicine* (ed. D. Skinner, A. Swain, R. Peyton, and C. Robertson, (pp. 498–504). Cambridge University Press.

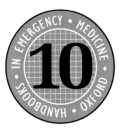

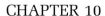

Neck and trunk wounds

Key points in neck and trunk wounds

Neck wounds

- Get senior help and secure the airway.
- Control bleeding by direct pressure.
- Do not explore these wounds in the A&E department.

Chest wounds

- Treat shock aggressively and get immediate surgical help.
- Tension pneumothorax: treat on clinical suspicion.
- Cover sucking chest wounds.
- Suspect cardiac tamponade in any penetrating wound near the heart.
- Use a blunt dissection technique through the 'triangle of safety' for chest drainage.

Abdominal wounds

- Treat shock aggressively and get immediate surgical help.
- Admit penetrating wounds.

Neck wounds

Open neck wounds are rare. Many are due to intentional self-harm. Management follows the routine of resuscitation, history, examination, investigation, and treatment.

Airway control

The airway is very much at risk in open injury. The pharynx (between the chin and the laryngeal prominence), the larynx, and the trachea are relatively superficial. Loss of normal anatomy and bleeding may seriously compromise the airway and also make it difficult to secure the airway by usual methods. IMMEDIATE SKILLED SENIOR HELP IS ESSENTIAL.

Patients may have adopted a position which keeps their airway open, so do not force them to lie down, as this might cause airway collapse.

If the patient is confused or unconscious them urgent action will be required. The route to secure the airway will depend on the skills available at the time. IMMEDIATE ACTION IS NEEDED. The options are:

1. **Oro-endotracheal intubation.** Prepare equipment and have good suction available. If inexperienced do not give muscle relaxants.
2. **Needle insufflation.** Percutaneous placement of a large-bore (14–12 gauge) cannula can 'buy time' while senior help arrives. The usual site of placement is through the cricothyroid membrane. If the larynx is injured then placement into the trachea is possible.
3. **A surgical airway.** Cricothyroidotomy is the preferred site in an adult provided the wound is above this level. An incision is made through the membrane and a cuffed endotracheal tube or tracheostomy tube is inserted. (Full details of these procedures are found in *The management of major trauma* by Robertson and Redmond, 1994.)

The main danger with all the surgical techniques is wrong positioning of the tube into the soft tissues around the larynx. If ventilation is difficult or massive subcutaneous surgical emphysema is noted check the tube's position.

Breathing

The proximity of the neck to the lung apices and the great vessels of the mediastinum may lead to pneumothorax/haemothorax. Look for these and treat as necessary (see below).

Haemorrhage control

> **Bleeding from neck wounds should be controlled by DIRECT PRESSURE. DO NOT ATTEMPT TO CLAMP BLEEDING VESSELS IN THE DEPTH OF THE WOUND.**

Two large-bore cannulae are placed, blood is taken for cross-matching, and fluid resuscitation is commenced.

AIR EMBOLUS may be caused by wounds of the large neck veins. Prevent negative pressure in the neck veins by ensuring the patient lies FLAT.

All significant neck wounds will require formal exploration, and should be referred to the appropriate in-patient team.

Chest wounds

- Introduction • Assessment • Tension pneumothorax
- Sucking chest wounds • Shock • Cardiac wounds
- Chest drainage

Introduction

Penetrating chest wounds are one of the few situations where minutes count. Stab wounds are the commonest cause of such injuries in the UK.

IF THE PATIENT IS SHOCKED THEN IMMEDIATE SURGICAL HELP IS REQUIRED.

Box 10.1 **Immediately life-threatening conditions**
- tension pneumothorax
- sucking chest wound
- massive haemothorax
- cardiac tamponade

Assessment

An accurate history should be obtained of the exact wounding mechanism. Check:

(1) the respiratory rate
(2) for the presence of dyspnoea
(3) chest movement—this is often the best way to detect pneumothorax
(4) for tracheal deviation and distended neck veins
(5) the percussion note and breath sounds

Cardiac tamponade should be suspected in any patient with a wound between the nipples anteriorly and the scapulae posteriorly. The neck veins may be distended, heart sounds will be muffled, the patient will show increasing signs of shock, and pulsus paradoxus will be marked.

Tension pneumothorax

This is a valve-like wound which is causing a continual leak of air into the pleural space, with a dangerous build-up in intrapleural pressure. This will collapse the lung, but will also cause a shift of the mediastinum, with kinking of the great veins, a reduction in cardiac return, and severe hypotension.

Diagnosis

- Respiratory distress
- Hypotension and shock
- Tracheal shift and distended neck veins
- Unequal chest movement
- Hyperresonance in percussion note
- Diminished breath sounds

Treatment TENSION PNEUMOTHORAX IS A CLINICAL DIAGNOSIS. Immediately insert a large-bore (14-gauge) cannula into the second intercostal space in the mid-clavicular line. Insert a formal chest drain.

Sucking chest wounds

Air will be drawn in through the wound during inspiration, leading to diminished air flow through the trachea and interfering with lung ventilation. The development of a tension pneumothorax is also a possibility. Treatment is to cover the wound with a dressing taped on three sides, leaving the fourth side free to allow air to escape. A chest drain is placed in the routine way (see p. 191)—it is NOT placed through the wound.

Shock

The commonest cause of shock in a penetrating trunk wound is hypovolaemia due to blood loss. However, tension pneumothorax and cardiac tamponade will present with shock. These rapidly lethal conditions must be excluded in chest and upper abdominal wounds.

Assessment The signs of shock (pallor, sweating, and restlessness) are better indicators of the shock state at this early stage than blood pressure. There is often a tachycardia and a low-volume pulse (beware: the pulse may be slow, especially in young and fit individuals). Check the neck veins, since venous distension in the presence of shock will indicate a tension pneumothorax or cardiac tamponade.

Treatment The surgical team is called immediately.

Venous access is secured using at least two 16-gauge cannulae, and blood is sent for cross-matching. Fluid replacement is begun using either a plasma expander, such as the gelatin solutions, or crystalloid solution. The rate will depend on the clinical response of the patient. The aim is to maintain the blood pressure between 60 and 90 mmHg systolic. The patient must be taken to theatre as quickly as possible for definitive haemorrhage control.

If haemothorax is the cause of the shock, then insert a chest drain. Note the loss of blood from the drain. An initial loss of greater than one litre or an ongoing loss of more than 200 ml per hour for four hours are indications for thoracotomy.

Immediate surgery is the best treatment for shocked patients with penetrating chest wounds.

Cardiac wounds

In any wound over the anterior part of the chest and upper abdomen damage to the heart must be expected and excluded. Penetrating wounds may damage the major cardiac chambers, valves, coronary arteries, or veins. The main problem is haemorrhage. This may cause a haemothorax or haemomediastinum. Immediate surgical intervention may be required.

The A&E management includes the normal care of the airway, breathing, and circulation, immediate surgical referral, and chest drainage.

Cardiac tamponade is described in detail, since immediate intervention may save the patient's life. It is the main indication for thoracotomy in the A&E department.

Cardiac tamponade is due to a wound of the heart causing haemorrhage into the pericardium. The non-distensible nature of the pericardium means that the external pressure on the heart rises, and this compresses the atria, reducing venous return, and thus reducing cardiac output. Continuing haemorrhage into the pericardium leads to ever-increasing pressure and profound shock.

Diagnosis
1. Consider tamponade as a possibility in every patient with a penetrating wound which may involve the heart.
2. Look for clinical signs of shock.
3. Look for distended neck veins and muffled heart sounds.
4. Pulsus paradoxus is a further indicator of tamponade, but the measurement of the difference in systolic blood pressures with inspiration and expiration may be very difficult.

Treatment. Speed is vital in the treatment of cardiac tamponade. If the patient is deteriorating urgent surgical help is essential, the patient requires immediate thoracotomy.

1. Call for immediate senior A&E, surgical, and anaesthetic assistance.
2. Secure two large-bore peripheral lines. Send blood for cross-matching. Cardiac output may be temporarily increased by elevating the right heart-filling pressure by giving a large intravenous bolus of fluid.
3. Make preparations for intubation/pericardiocentesis/thoracotomy.

Immediate thoracotomy is the treatment of choice for haemopericardium causing cardiac tamponade. Pericardiocentesis may relieve the intrapericardial pressure temporarily while surgical assistance arrives.

The technique of pericardiocentesis is demonstrated in Figure 10.1.

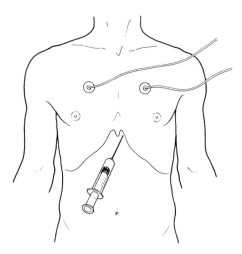

Fig. 10.1 • Pericardiocentesis. Observe ECG while performing this procedure.

If the patient is stable and there is diagnostic doubt then urgent ultrasound in the A&E department is the best investigation.

Chest drainage

Many penetrating chest injuries will require placement of a chest drain. This is not always an easy procedure at three a.m. with a drunk hypoxic patient. The procedure is described in Box 10.2, and illustrated in Figure 10.2.

Box 10.2 Insertion of intercostal chest drain

1. Identify the 'triangle of safety', whose surface markings are:
   - lateral border of pectoralis major
   - mid-axillary line
   - nipple level (5th intercostal space)
2. Prepare and drape the chest.
3. Remove the trocar from the chest drain and clamp the proximal end.
4. Anaesthetize the skin and deeper layers, to the level of rib periosteum.
5. Make a 2–3 cm transverse incision, followed by blunt dissection with curved scissors, keeping just above the rib.
6. Penetrate the parietal pleura, and insert a finger into the pleural cavity to confirm that there are no underlying organs or adherent lung tissue.
7. Using your finger, guide the chest drain into the pleural cavity. *Do not use a blind technique with a trocar.*
8. Connect the drain to the underwater-seal apparatus and remove the clamp.
9. Secure the tube in place and obtain a chest X-ray.

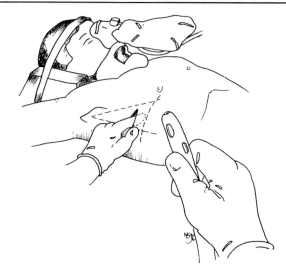

Fig. 10.2 • Insertion of intercostal chest drain.

Abdominal wounds

- **Introduction** • **Resuscitation** • **Diagnosis**
- **Surgical referral**

Introduction

Aetiology. Blunt trauma is the commonest cause for serious intra-abdominal injury, but stab wounds are increasing in incidence in the United Kingdom. The function of the A&E department in the management of such injury is:

1. *Resuscitation.* Assessment and control of the airway, breathing, and circulation.

2. *Immediate surgical referral.* The more unstable the patient the earlier the surgical and anaesthetic teams should be involved.

3. *Diagnosis.* Have a high index of suspicion for intra-abdominal injury. The history of the mechanism of injury is often the sole early indicator of intra-abdominal problems.

Clinical signs may well be absent or hard to interpret, especially if there are other injuries.

4. *Assessment* and the initial management of other injuries. In blunt trauma it is rare for the abdomen to be the only area injured.

5. *To co-ordinate resuscitation, investigations, and treatment, and to formulate management plans.* The involvement of many surgical teams may cause some confusion and lack of direction. It is essential that the overall condition of the patient is appreciated and definite plans are made and carried out.

Resuscitation

In isolated abdominal wounds the airway is not a problem. Breathing may well be affected owing to the close proximity of the lower chest and upper abdomen. Pneumothorax and haemothorax should be excluded.

The major resuscitation problem is often that of shock.

It is important to recognize the signs of shock at an early stage (see p. 21). Establish two large-bore intravenous lines and take blood for urgent cross-matching. Immediate surgical assistance is essential. The need for fluid replacement will depend on the degree of shock. If the blood pressure is maintained at 90 mmHg or above then no fluid may be needed PROVIDED THAT IMMEDIATE SURGERY CAN BE CARRIED OUT TO STOP THE HAEMORRHAGE.

Rarely, shock may be due to cardiac wounds so check the neck veins.

Pass a naso-gastric tube (assuming there is no major facial injury).

Pass a urinary catheter (assuming that the wound does not involve the perineum and there are no signs of urethral injury such as blood at the urethral meatus).

Diagnosis

Obtain a clear history of the method of wounding. The number and types of organ injury are very different in gunshot wounds and stab wounds.

Examine the whole of the trunk paying special attention to the back and perineum. Note all wounds, measure the wounds and record any other features surrounding the wound such as bruising or burning. Palpate for tenderness and percussion tenderness. Perform a rectal examination.

Investigations must include a chest X-ray (erect if possible). This will exclude pneumothorax or haemothorax and may show gas under the diaphragm. In those patients who cannot sit up a lateral decubitus X-ray is invaluable in detecting free intraperitoneal air. In gunshot wounds plain abdominal films should be taken to show the number and path of bullets.

Urine should be checked for blood.

Intravenous urography is indicated if renal injury is suspected. It is essential to know if the patient has two functioning kidneys prior to surgery for severe renal injury.

IF THERE ARE SIGNS OF INTRAPERITONEAL INJURY THEN OTHER INVESTIGATIONS ARE NOT NECESSARY. LAPAROTOMY IS INDICATED.

Ultrasound is increasingly used in the diagnosis of abdominal injury. It will show the presence of free fluid and delineate haematomas in or around the solid organs.

Peritoneal lavage is highly sensitive in revealing intraperitoneal pathology. It is invasive and local policy regarding its use should be agreed.

Computerized tomography is the best method for imaging the retroperitoneal structures such as the pancreas.

Other injury. Even penetrating wounds cause damage to other areas outside the confines of the abdomen. Chest injury is common, since the chest shares the 'same space' as the upper abdominal organs. It is separated from them only by a thin sheet of muscle, which is easily penetrated.

Stabbings and gunshot wounds may be multiple. A full examination of the whole patient must be performed (REMEMBER THE BACK).

Surgical referral

In some conditions it is expected that patients should be fully investigated before referral is made. This should NOT be done in abdominal injuries.

> ***EARLY SURGICAL REFERRAL IS MANDATORY.* There is no sense in proceeding with aggressive fluid replacement if it is pouring into the peritoneal cavity. Early surgical intervention saves lives.**

Further reading

1. Robertson, C. and Redmond, A.D. (1994). *The management of major trauma.* Oxford University Press.
2. Skinner, D., Driscoll, P., and Earlam, R. (1996). *ABC of major trauma.* British Medical Journal Publications, London.
3. Bickell, W.H., Wall, M.J., Pepe, P.E., Martin, R.R., Ginger, V.E., Allen, M.K., and Mattox, K.L. (1994). Immediate versus delayed fluid resuscitation for hypotensive patients with penetrating torso injuries. *New England Journal of Medicine,* **331**, 1105–9.

PART 4
Burns management

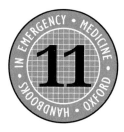

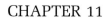

General principles

Introduction
Epidemiology

Minor burns and scalds are everyday problems in the A&E department. It is estimated that 150000 new patients will attend A&E departments each year with a burn injury. The follow up and aftercare of many small burns will take place in the department.

Serious burns are less common than minor ones but they are an important cause of mortality and morbidity. In England and Wales during 1996, 442 people died from the effects of fire. Each year, 15000 patients require admission to hospital.

The early care of the seriously burned patient The direct effect of the burn is only one component of the injuries of a seriously burned patient, and the assessment and treatment of pulmonary complications, poisoning from fumes, and blast injury will be discussed.

Agents causing burning

- **Wet heat** • **Dry heat** • **Chemicals** • **Electricity**
- **Radiation**

Wet heat Although most scalds will result in superficial skin loss, boiling water from a domestic kettle will cause full-thickness skin loss in a few seconds. Steam, especially superheated steam, will cause greater damage, owing to the release of the latent heat of vaporization. Boiling fat is at a higher temperature than water, and deeper damage results.

Scalds are the commonest type of burn injury presenting to A&E departments, especially in the young.

Dry heat Direct burns from a flame, often from matches or cigarettes, are the second most common cause of burns. If the clothing catches fire, the resulting burns are always serious. Contact with hot domestic appliances, such as irons or ovens, is a common source of minor burns. Although often fairly small in size, they are usually deep burns. Molten metal burns are usually full-thickness; they are becoming less common as the metal-working industries scale down.

Chemicals The severity of the burn will depend on the type of chemical, its concentration, and the contact time. It is essential that all traces of the chemical are removed by copious lavage.

Cement. This causes one of the commonest deep chemical burns. Whilst working with cement, some may penetrate the clothing, or dust may enter the boots. If the cement then comes into contact with water, the lime will produce a burn injury. This will go unnoticed by the patient until the clothing is removed, giving the worst possible circumstance: a concentrated solution of caustic chemical which is left in contact with the skin for a considerable time.

Hydrofluoric acid. This acid is used in metal processing and cleaning. It penetrates the skin readily, and goes on to cause a great deal of tissue destruction. These burns are treated with the usual copious lavage, and then with the application of calcium gluconate gel. Regional intravenous infusion of calcium gluconate should be considered in burns of the forearm or hand if topical treatment fails (seek advice).

Phenol. If the burn involves a large area it may allow enough systemic uptake of the phenol to give rise to renal failure.

Electricity The depth of the burn is dependent on the energy transfer to the tissues. This will be greater with high-voltage sources, or if the skin resistance is low owing to the presence of moisture. Contact time may be increased if the current causes tetanic contraction of the muscles. There may be relative sparing of the skin, but with gross damage to deeper tissues.

Most domestic-supply burns give small punctate deep burns at the entry point. The passage of the current across the chest (as when the entry point is in an upper limb and the earth is the ground) may cause fatal cardiac arrhythmias.

When the hand grasps an electric fire the combination of direct heat and electricity usually causes a severe burn.

High-voltage supply will cause severe and extensive burns with massive tissue destruction.

Radiation The commonest burns of this nature are the burns caused by exposure to sunlight or on sunbeds. These are always superficial, but can be extensive and are often very painful. Full-body sunburn may require admission.

'Welder's flash' is a radiation burn of the eye. The light radiation from the welding arc causes small punctate burns of the corneal epithelium (see the section on eye wounds in Chapter 9, p. 237).

Radiation burns caused by ionizing radiation are uncommon in A&E practice. The commonest source of these burns is probably iatrogenic, resulting from the radiotherapy of tumours, but these patients seldom present to the A&E department.

Estimation of burn depth

- **History** • **Erythema** • **Superficial partial thickness**
- **Deep partial thickness** • **Full thickness**

The depth of burn will depend on:

(1) the *intensity* of the burning agent (or concentration in chemical burns)
(2) the *time* the burning agent is in contact with the skin

A full-thickness burn may be caused by brief contact with molten metal, but may equally well be caused by prolonged contact with a moderately hot central heating radiator.

Initial treatment is based on the estimation of burn depth. This is described according to the level of the skin involved. The various levels of skin damage are shown in Figure 11.1, along with the clinical features of each type of burn.

Erythema alone causes no skin loss, and will heal with no scarring.

A *superficial partial-thickness* burn will have thin-walled

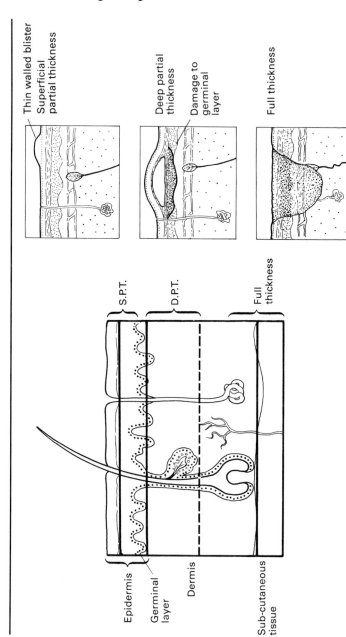

Fig. 11.1 • Depth of burn and clinical correlation.

blisters. The skin is red, weeping, and tender. This burn involves the upper layers of the epidermis, but, since it leaves the germinal layer intact, will heal quickly with little scarring.

A *deep partial-thickness* burn will have a whiter appearance than a more superficial burn. The hair follicles may be apparent as small, punctate red areas. As the germinal layer is lost, healing will occur by migration of epidermal cells from the skin appendages and wound edges. Healing will be slow, and there may be problems resulting from scarring and contractures. Further progression of the depth of the burn may occur if the wound becomes dessicated or infected. If the area is large then skin grafting is the treatment of choice.

Full-thickness burns appear hard and leathery. Coagulated vessels may be seen. Sensation is absent. Such burns will only heal from the skin edges, and heal slowly and with problems of scarring and contracture. Skin grafting is required.

Estimation of burn size

- **Exclude erythema** • **Use body chart**
- **'Patient's hand' method** • **'Rule of nines'**
- **'Rule of fives'**

Doctors who have little experience with severely burned patients tend to OVERESTIMATE the size of the burn.

Erythema. Do NOT include areas of erythema in the calculation of the burn area. These should be noted separately.

Use **body charts** to increase the accuracy of estimates (Fig. 11.2). Draw the extent of the burn on the chart and then simply add up the percentages.

Small areas may be estimated by using the **patient's hand** as a guide. The hand with the fingers extended and adducted is approximately 1 per cent of the patient's body area (Fig. 11.3).

The traditional method of area estimation is the '**Rule of nines**'. Figure 11.4 shows how the body is divided into sections, giving the percentage of body area in each section.

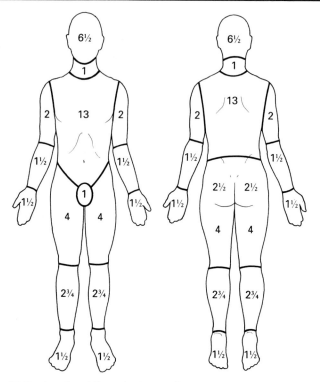

Fig. 11.2 • Lund and Browder burns chart.

This method is inaccurate for infants; Figure 11.4 shows the '**Rule of fives**' applicable to the young.

Principles of treatment of the burn wound

- **Remove burning agent** • **Asepsis** • **Exclusion**
- **Exposure** • **Excision and grafting**
- **Tetanus prophylaxis** • **No routine antibiotics**
- **Referral**

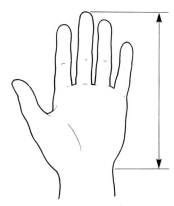

Fig. 11.3 . The patient's hand represents 1% of the total body surface area.

'Rule of nines' (adults)	'Rule of fives' (infants)
9 Head	20 Head
9 Each upper limb	10 Each upper limb
18 Front trunk	20 Front trunk
18 Back trunk	20 Back trunk
18 Each lower limb	10 Each lower limb
1 Perineum	

Fig. 11.4 . 'Rule of nines' for adults and 'Rule of fives' for infants.

The treatment needed will depend on the depth of the burn, its size, and the part of the body involved.

Remove burning agent All traces of the burning agent are removed. In chemical burns the affected area must be washed with large volumes of water. However, if dry powder or crystals are present these should be brushed off before lavage.

Asepsis Most burns will heal if infection is avoided. Strict aseptic routine is used in the A&E department. If a burn is infected then the healing time may be prolonged. A severe infection may convert a partial-thickness injury into a full-thickness injury.

Exclusion The exclusion of infection by the application of a dressing is the mainstay of the treatment of most small burns. The method is described in detail on p. 233. Soiled dressings are changed, or else bacteria may gain easy entry to the burn.

Exposure The face, the perineum, and some parts of the trunk are hard to dress adequately. In these areas the burn wound may be left open. This will normally require admission, except with minor, superficial burns of the face.

Excision and grafting Almost all full-thickness burns will require excision of the dead skin and skin grafting. Large, deep partial-thickness burns will also require such skilled care. These procedures are not normally carried out in the A&E department.

Tetanus prophylaxis As in all wounds, adequate tetanus immunization must be given.

No routine antibiotics Routine prophylactic antibiotics are NOT usually required. Some patients may present some days after burning with signs of infection. Antibiotics are needed if there is evidence of spreading infection such as cellulitis. The commonest infecting organisms will be the beta-haemolytic streptococcus and *Staphylococcus aureus*. Children may develop toxic shock syndrome with infected burns. Medicated dressings (e.g. Bactigras) are advised as prophylaxis. Flucloxacillin or erythromycin are recommended for the treatment of INFECTED burn wounds.

Referral Most minor scalds and burns are treated by the A&E department. Serious burns and large deep partial-thickness and full-thickness burns will need referral. It may be difficult at the time of initial presentation to decide the depth of a burn. If the area is relatively small (1–5 per cent) then the wound may be dressed and the patient referred for a senior opinion. Take greater care with burns of important areas such as the eyes or hands. Have a low threshold for referring such burns.

> **Box 11.1 Criteria for immediate senior opinion/referral**
>
> Burns involving more than 10% of total body surface area (less in a child).
> Full-thickness burns of more than 1% total body surface area.
> Serious burns of hands, eyes, or perineum.
> Burns involving the airway.
> Significant smoke inhalation.

Systemic effects of burn injury

- Circulation • Kidney • Heat loss
- Immune system

Circulation

There are obvious losses from weeping areas of partial-thickness burns, but in addition burn injury causes widespread changes in vascular permeability throughout the body. This leads to loss of plasma from the vascular system and hypovolaemic shock.

Although the initial loss is of plasma, red cells are also destroyed, either directly in the burned area or by later haemolysis.

Shock must be diagnosed and treated aggressively in the A&E department.

Kidney

Acute renal failure is a serious complication of large burns. Hypovolaemia and the normal responses to shock greatly reduce renal perfusion. The release of haemoglobin from haemolysed red cells or myoglobin from damaged muscle adds to the insult to the kidney.

The assessment of renal function should begin in the A&E department. The seriously burned patient should be catheterized, and the urine volume measured hourly. The urine should be examined for the presence of haem pigments. Blood samples should be sent for baseline urea, electrolytes, and osmolality estimations.

Heat loss

Severely burned patients, particularly children, are liable to lose heat; blister fluid evaporates and normal capillary control is lost in the damaged skin. If the burn area is large, cold water soaks should NOT be applied; there is a significant risk of inducing hypothermia, especially in children.

Immune system

Large burn injuries cause severe depression of the immune system. This renders the patient very susceptible to infection. The prevention of infection should begin in the A&E department. Gloves should be used when handling the patient. The wounds should be covered with sterile dressings. Unnecessary invasive procedures, such as routine central venous cannulation, should be avoided.

Other injuries in burns patients

- **Trauma** • **Smoke inhalation**
- **Carbon monoxide poisoning** • **Cyanide poisoning**
- **Blast injury**

The burn may be only one aspect of the injury sustained by a patient. More people involved in house fires die as a result of carbon monoxide poisoning than as a result of burns. Similarly, a burn will be only one component of the injury sustained in an explosion, where wounds may be caused by debris, and the blast wave may also cause severe damage to internal organs.

Some of these other injuries will now be considered.

Trauma

Patients may have suffered severe injury in trying to escape from a fire, jumping from a window for example. A full examination of the patient must be performed, or such injuries may be overlooked.

Smoke inhalation

The lungs may suffer direct heat injury from inhaled gases, or a chemical pneumonitis from toxic fumes. Eighty-five per cent of patients suffering from smoke inhalation will have been exposed to a fire in a confined space. The frequency of symptoms and signs of this syndrome are given in Table 11.1.

If significant smoke inhalation is suspected then the patient should be admitted and closely observed both clinically and by serial blood–gas measurement.

Carbon monoxide poisoning

This is the leading cause of death from all poisonings. It is especially common in fires in confined areas, and it is often the combination of toxic fumes and carbon monoxide that causes fatalities in house fires.

For this reason it should be *routine* to measure the arterial levels of carbon monoxide in all patients with severe burns caused by fire.

Table 11.1 . Frequency of symptoms and signs in patients with smoke inhalation

Sign/symptom	Percentage of patients
Exposed to a fire in an enclosed space	85
Respiratory symptoms	75
Respiratory signs	73
Decreased conscious level	65
Soot in sputum	40
Perioral burning	30
Hoarseness	30

Carbon monoxide has an affinity for the haem group which is 96 times greater than that of oxygen. Thus the oxygen-carrying capacity of the blood is greatly reduced. The haem group is also part of the cytochrome p450 system, an essential part of cellular aerobic respiration. The carbon monoxide will remain bound to this system, even when blood levels have fallen to normal. This interruption of normal cellular metabolism will continue to cause damage.

The clinical presentation will depend on the extent of the exposure. In a severe case the patient is unconscious, and often has a rapid, bounding pulse.

With lesser degrees of exposure the patient may have a spectrum of symptoms ranging from no abnormality to alteration in conscious level and focal neurological defects, most commonly of the extrapyramidal system. The lack of oxygen-carrying capacity may also cause ischaemic symptoms. If there are pre-existing vascular lesions, such as coronary artery stenoses, this might lead to myocardial infarction.

High-flow oxygen therapy is the mainstay of treatment. Hyperbaric oxygen therapy should be considered in the presence of:

- Carboxyhaemoglobin level >40%
- History of unconsciousness
- Cardiac complications
- Persistent neurological deficit or coma
- Pregnancy

If serious injuries are also present, transfer of the patient for hyperbaric oxygen therapy may be impractical.

Cyanide poisoning

Modern furniture containing polyurethane and nylon gives off hydrogen cyanide when burnt. The signs of cyanide poisoning are predominantly neurological, with headache, dizziness, and fits. There may be tachypnoea and hypertension in the early stages of poisoning, but severe poisoning will lead to a slowing of the respiratory rate and hypotension.

There are no unique features which will indicate cyanide poisoning, and the diagnosis will be missed unless the doctor is aware of this possibility.

The treatment is controversial, and in the context of the severely burned patient it would be wise to seek advice before embarking on complex treatment of cyanide poisoning in the A&E department (see p. 226).

Blast injury

An explosion will produce *direct physical injury* as fragments penetrate the body, or as the patient is thrown by the blast or crushed by falling debris. The heat from the explosion will produce *thermal burns*. Finally, the patient will sustain *blast damage*. The explosion will produce high-energy sound waves, which tend to give up energy at the interface between media of differing density. In the body this occurs at the interface between body fluid and air, so the structures most involved in blast injury are the air-containing organs, the lungs and the bowel. Patients may present with deafness due to middle ear damage.

In the context of a patient who is badly burned as a result of an explosion the possibility of blast injury should be kept in mind. Ventilatory support may be required for lung damage, and laparotomy may be needed for abdominal complications.

Further reading

1. Monafo, W. (1996). Initial management of burns. *New England Journal of Medicine*, **21**, 1581–6.
2. Dougherty, W. and Waxman, K. (1996). The complexities of managing severe burns with associated trauma. *Surgical Clinics of North America*, **76**, 923–51.
3. Langford, R.M. and Armstrong, R.F. (1989). Algorithm for managing injury from smoke inhalation. *British Medical Journal*, **299**, 902–5.
4. Muir, I.F.K., Barclay, T.L., and Settle, J.A.D. (1987). *Burns and their treatment*. Butterworth, London.
5. Swain, A.H., Azadian, B.S., Wakely, C.J., and Shakespeare, P.G.

(1987). Management of blisters in minor burns. *British Medical Journal*, **295**, 181.

6. Robertson, C. (1996). *Management of severe burns.* In *ABC of major trauma* (ed. D. Skinner, P. Driscoll, and R. Earlam) pp 118, 123. British Medical Journal Publications, London.

7. Ryan, J.M. (1997). Burns and scalds. In *Cambridge textbook of accident and emergency medicine* (ed. D. Skinner, A. Swain, R. Peyton, and C. Robertson), pp. 721–32 Cambridge University Press.

8. Graudins, A., Burns, M.J., and Aaron, C.K. (1997). Regional intravenous infusion of calcium gluconate for hydrofluoric acid burns of the upper extremity. *Annals of Emergency Medicine*, **30**, 604–7.

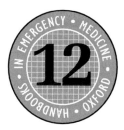

Serious burns

Key points in serious burns

- Senior help required.
- Use sterile gloves and technique.
- Remove all clothing/all the burning agent.
- Look for signs of upper airway burning.
- Perform early endotracheal intubation if airway is at risk.
- Insert two large-bore intravenous cannulae.
- Resuscitate using plasma if possible.
- Look for signs of smoke inhalation.
- Blood tests—haematocrit, osmolarity, gases, carbon monoxide.
- Insert urinary catheter/naso-gastric tube.
- Full examination assessing—burn area
  —burn depth
  —other injury
  —medical problems
- Seek advice from local burns unit early.
- Transfer patient only when stable.

Definition

A serious burn is present if one of the following conditions are met:

1. There are burns involving more than 15 per cent of the body surface area in an adult, or more than 10 per cent in a child (excluding erythema).
2. There are full-thickness burns of more than 5 per cent of body area.
3. There are burns involving the airway.
4. There are deep burns in especially important areas (e.g. eyes or hands).

Resuscitation

- **Remove burning agent** • **Airway** • **Breathing**
- **Circulation**

Remove all traces of the burning agent

This is especially important in chemical burns. All clothing must be removed.

Airway

Secure early in severely burned patients. Burns of the airway cause local oedema, and this may progress rapidly to complete upper airway obstruction.

Assessment Check the nares and mouth for any signs of burning (coughing, hoarseness, pain on breathing or swallowing, singeing of nasal hair, erythema or blistering of the mouth, soot in the nose or mouth). If these signs are present in a badly burned patient call for immediate senior help.

Stridor is a late sign. DO NOT WAIT for stridor to appear before considering endotracheal intubation.

Treatment If the airway appears to be uninjured then give high-flow oxygen, humidified if possible.

> If there are signs that suggest possible airway
> damage early endotracheal intubation is
> ESSENTIAL.

Breathing

Lung damage may occur as a result of direct thermal damage to small airways or chemical pneumonitis. Hypoventilation may be caused by carbon monoxide or cyanide poisoning. All these problems may be found in a patient involved in a fire in a confined space (e.g. a house fire).

Full-thickness burns of the chest wall may make chest movement very difficult and may interfere with lung ventilation.

Assessment Note the depth, rate, and ease of respiration.

Treatment In this phase of management the only treatment possible is to secure the airway and supply high-flow oxygen, with humidification if possible.

If full-thickness chest burns are restricting ventilation urgent escharotomy is required. This is done simply by splitting the full-thickness area with a scalpel. The procedure will be pain-free because of the destruction of the cutaneous nerves by the burn.

Circulation

Assessment Look for evidence of shock (a pale, sweaty, clammy, anxious patient). Note the pulse. Check capillary return.

Treatment Secure venous access immediately. The usual sites for placing cannulae may actually be involved in the burn. Fluid loss results in shock and peripheral vasoconstriction, further adding to the difficulty.

In such circumstances it is essential to place a large-bore cannula (at least 16-gauge) into any available vein. The following action plan is recommended:

1. Use a *large arm vein*, the antecubital fossa, or the cephalic vein at the wrist. It is preferable to use a vein in an area that is not burned; however, it is permissible to use a vein in the burned area if no other is available.
2. Send for *senior help.*
3. Use the *external jugular vein* in an area that is not burned.
4. *Cut down* on the arm veins or long saphenous vein at the ankle.
5. The *femoral vein*. To achieve adequate flow rates a large-bore cannula will be required, inserted using the Seldinger technique.
6. The *internal jugular/subclavian veins.*

Children The help of a senior A&E doctor, or an experienced paediatrician or anaesthetist is essential. If senior help is not immediately available, try to secure venous access. However, do not damage all potential infusion sites — confine the attempt to one limb. If venous access is not obtained after two or three tries, then more experienced help is vital.

In infants the *scalp* veins may be used. In preschool children the *external jugular* is often used. If no other access is possible then *intra-osseous infusion* may be life-saving.

Undress During the process of resuscitation all clothing will have been removed. Water lavage is indicated for chemical or some radiation burns (see p. 202), but in other burns large areas should be temporarily wrapped in cling-film.

Assessment: history

- **How? Where? When?**   • **Tetanus/allergies/medication**
- **Other symptoms** • **Past medical history**

Ask the questions HOW? WHERE? and WHEN? The patient may be unable to give an adequate history, so it is essential to gain as much information as possible from the ambulance personnel.

How?

When clothing has been on fire the burn is often deep. Similarly, petrol burns are often full-thickness. High-voltage electrical burns cause massive tissue destruction. Many chemicals cause deep burning, especially lime (most commonly as part of cement).

Ascertain the duration of exposure to the burning agent.

Is there anything in the history to suggest the inhalation of smoke? a fall? a blast?

Any first aid measures which have been performed should be documented.

Where?

Certain accident locations may give pointers to the possible complications. In house fires there is a high likelihood that the patient will have inhaled smoke. This may lead to upper-airway burning, carbon monoxide poisoning, or chemical pneumonitis (or all three). In industrial chemical accidents the exact composition of the chemicals must be sought, since they may have systemic toxic effects as well as causing burning.

When?

Most severe burns reach hospital quickly, but it is important to know the time since burning in order to calculate the fluid requirements.

Tetanus, allergies, medication

As in all wounds the tetanus immunization status of the patient, any allergy, and any medications must be noted.

Other symptoms

The degree of pain may give some indication of the depth of the burn. It is important to ensure that the patient is given adequate analgesia.

Elicit such symptoms as hoarseness, pain on swallowing/breathing, and difficulty in breathing.

Past medical history

Some serious burns are a direct consequence of another illness (e.g. collapse into a hot bath as a result of myocardial ischaemia), and the presence of symptoms which seem unrelated to the burn must be noted and further assessed.

A large burn causes very great changes in the fluid balance and the body's metabolism. The mortality from burns is increased in the presence of other serious medical illness. Pre-existing cardiac, renal, and metabolic disease (especially diabetes) or alcohol abuse (acute or chronic) must be noted.

Assessment: examination and investigation

- Vital signs • Head-to-toe survey
- Estimation of burn area/depth • Investigations

Vital signs

Pulse, blood pressure, respiratory rate, and Glasgow Coma Score are recorded.

Continuous electrocardiograph monitoring is commenced.

Head-to-toe survey

It will be tempting to proceed directly to the assessment of the burn, but if this is done other burned areas and other injuries may be missed. A full 'head-to-toe' examination must be performed.

Pay particular attention to the face, looking for erythema or blistering of the nose, lips, or mouth. Note the presence of soot in the nose or mouth. Look carefully at the eyes. If there is any suggestion of corneal damage fluorescein must be instilled at some stage to assess the extent of burning.

On examination of the chest note the signs of any other injuries, and listen carefully to the breath sounds. At this early stage the presence of any abnormal sounds indicates significant smoke inhalation.

Examine the abdomen, pelvis, perineum and limbs for any associated injury. Log-roll the patient to examine the back and the spine.

In burns of an extremity examine the circulation distal to the burn. In circumferential full-thickness burns contraction of the eschar may result in a tourniquet-like effect. This must be recognized, and the patient must be referred for immediate escharotomy.

Estimation of burn area/depth

Use the methods outlined earlier (see p. 205) to estimate the percentage of the body area involved in the burn. Remember simple erythema is NOT included in the estimation. Use special burn charts to improve accuracy and also to provide a good diagrammatic record.

The burn depth is estimated by the appearance of the burn wound and sensory function (sensitivity to pin-prick).

Investigations

During the initial resuscitation blood samples should have been taken for *urgent cross-matching*.

Haematology. A haemoglobin concentration, haematocrit, white cell count, and platelet count should be performed. The haematocrit is of special importance, since it is a good method of monitoring the adequacy of fluid replacement. In the first few hours after the burn these values may be relatively normal, and therefore should not be used as a guide to INITIAL fluid therapy.

Biochemistry. Urea, creatinine, electrolyte concentrations, and plasma osmolality should be measured, and baseline values noted. Any decline in renal function can then be monitored.

Urine. An indwelling urinary catheter is placed. The residual urine volume is noted and tested for free haemoglobin and myoglobin, and urine osmolality is measured.

An arterial blood sample must be sent for estimation of blood gas tensions and blood hydrogen ion concentration (or pH). The blood carboxyhaemoglobin should also be measured. Note that pulse oximetry cannot be used reliably in this situation. The presence of carboxyhaemoglobin renders

> **The hourly urine volume is the easiest method of estimating response to fluid therapy, and measurements should be commenced as early as possible.**

pulse oximetry inaccurate—the readings will be artificially high.

The results of routine oxygen tension require careful interpretation, since most blood gas analysers will measure the DISSOLVED oxygen in the blood and the haemoglobin saturation is CALCULATED, correcting for temperature and acid-base status. This calculation assumes normal haemoglobin binding.

> **If there is a high percentage of carboxyhaemoglobin then this will mean much less actual oxygen carriage than that which is calculated.**

Pulmonary function. If the patient can co-operate simple pulmonary function tests (such as for peak expiratory flow rate) should be carried out.

Radiology. An erect chest radiograph should be requested. In the early stages of chemical pneumonitis this radiograph is often NORMAL.

Further radiographs may be required if indicated by the history or by clinical examination.

Treatment

- Airway and breathing • Which fluid?
- How much fluid? • Treatment of the burn area
- Drugs • Carbon monoxide and cyanide poisoning
- Referral and transfer

Airway and breathing

If there are indications of upper airway burns then it is best to call for skilled help to pass an endotracheal tube. There should be no delay in carrying out this procedure, since laryngeal oedema progressing to complete respiratory obstruction may occur suddenly.

If there are no worries about the airway then high-flow oxygen is given (humidified if possible). Consider escharotomy in large full-thickness burns of the chest.

Which fluid?

'Replace like with like' is good rule of thumb to decide the type of fluid therapy to use after fluid loss.

In burns the exudate approaches the protein content of plasma (blister fluid 50 g/litre, plasma 65 g/litre.) The logical fluid replacement is therefore plasma.

There is great debate about the best fluid to give during the initial treatment of all forms of shock, and there is controversy in the treatment of burns shock. However, the use of plasma in the form of PPF (plasma protein fraction) is both safe and effective in the severely burned patient. This method will be described in detail. Alternatives include other colloids, such as the gelatin solutions, or starch solutions, or even simple electrolyte solutions. Each burns unit may have preferences, and these should be known to local A&E departments.

How much fluid?

There are many formulae which may be used to calculate the amounts of fluid required in a burns patient. It is vital to realize that these only give an *approximate guide* to the fluid requirements. Many other factors, such as the patient's age, or a previous history of heart disease or renal disease, may alter these requirements. The commonest formula used is that of Muir and Barclay, which is as follows:

The patient weight is in kilograms and the area of burn is expressed as a percentage of the total body area, and this gives the amount of plasma in MILLILITRES to be infused during the first four hours from burning.

Box 12.1 **Muir and Barclay formula for plasma replacement in a burns patient**

$$\text{ml OF } PLASMA = \frac{(\% \text{ AREA BURNED} \times PATIENT \text{ Wt})}{2}$$

This fluid is given in the first 4 hours from burning.

For example, if a *70 kg* adult sustains *30 per cent* burns and arrives in the A&E department *2 hours* after the burn then the initial fluid requirement will be:

$$\frac{(70 \times 30)}{2} = 1050 \text{ ml of plasma.}$$

Therefore approximately 1 litre of plasma will be required during the first TWO hours of the infusion, as two hours have already elapsed since the time of burning.

Such formulae can only act as an initial guide to fluid requirements. Note that this formula is a guide to the volume of fluid needed to *replace* the burn losses—in addition the patient will require normal *maintenance* fluids. The response of the patient to the fluid is the best guide to continuing requirements, and the patient should be monitored regularly by clinical examination and hourly urinary output. Once the patient is admitted other parameters, such as the haematocrit and urine osmolality, are used to monitor progress.

Treatment of the burn area

The first aid treatment is to remove all clothing and ensure complete removal of the burning agent. In extensive burns the use of cling-film to wrap the area is recommended. The use of large quantities of cold water-soaked sheets will make nursing difficult and lead to hypothermia.

The use of urgent escharotomy for constricting chest and circumferential limb wounds has been mentioned above.

Some burns will requires specific treatment, as suggested in Chapter 13 on minor burns (pp. 229–238).

Drugs

Analgesia Burning and scalding are terrifying experiences for patients and their families, and often for the staff that have to deal with the early treatment of the patient. There is pressure to use large doses of analgesia before anything else is done in these patients. Many burns are extremely painful, but also many severe burns are relatively pain-free. Once the initial resuscitation and assessment have been completed then analgesia should be given. The best way to give this is by small intravenous boluses of opiate. This method enables the response to be measured, but the respiratory rate and blood pressure can also be monitored.

Tetanus toxoid Tetanus toxoid and immunoglobulin should be given if indicated (see p. 104).

Antibiotics Prophylactic antibiotics should not be given routinely to severely burned patients.

Carbon monoxide and cyanide poisoning

Poisoning should be suspected in all seriously burned patients.

Carbon monoxide poisoning is treated with high-flow oxygen therapy. Consider seeking advice on hyperbaric oxygen treatment (Duty surgeon Commander, HMS *Portsmouth*, 01705 768 034.).

Cyanide poisoning treatment is dependent on the clinical state of the patient. In the unconscious patient with deteriorating blood pressure and respiratory rate secure the airway and ventilate with 100 per cent oxygen.

If cyanide poisoning is only *suspected* then give *10 ml of 3 per cent sodium nitrite solution* intravenously over 10 minutes. Then give 50 ml of 25 per cent sodium thiosulphate solution over 10 minutes.

If cyanide poisoning is *certain* then give *20 ml of 1.5 per cent dicobalt edetate* solution over 1 minute.

If the patient is conscious and cardiovascularly stable then supportive measures only are indicated.

Referral and transfer

The facility to which the patient is admitted will depend on a number of factors. If patients are severely shocked or require mechanical ventilation then they will require the facilities and the expertise of the staff in either an intensive care unit or a burns unit.

> **Transferring a critically ill patient some distance is a dangerous undertaking, and it is essential to resuscitate the patient in the receiving hospital and then transfer a stable patient.**

The management of the patient should be discussed at the earliest possible stage with the staff of the nearest burns unit. A management plan may then be formulated, and the expertise of the burns unit will have been involved as early as possible.

Criteria for transfer Only rough guidance can be given, since the criteria for admission will vary between burns units. Assess the patient, perform initial resuscitation and treatment, and then discuss the case with the surgical team and the local burns unit.

Burns of greater than 25–30 per cent may require admission to the burns unit. Other factors such as age, other injuries, or complications must also be taken into account in deciding whether to transfer.

Deep burns of more than 5 per cent of the body area and deep burns involving the hands or face will probably require transfer to a burns unit at some stage. The less severely burned will probably be treated on the general surgical wards.

The burns may be of such severity, and the patient so elderly that there is little likelihood of survival. Various formulae exist to estimate the chance of survival of an individual patient. However, the decision not to treat a severely burned patient should not be taken by an inexperienced junior doctor.

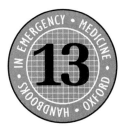

Minor burns

Key points in minor burns

- History—some burning agents will indicate the probability of deep/full-thickness burns.
- Depth of burn.
- Thin-walled blisters; red, weeping skin; intact sensation—superficial partial-thickness.
- Thick-walled blisters, white skin with red punctate areas, sensation intact/blunted—deep partial-thickness.
- White/brown, leathery skin, sensation absent—full-thickness.
- Special care burns: hand, eye, face, perineum.

Treatment

- Clean using aseptic technique.
- Blisters—leave intact or aspirate: do not deroof.
- Dressing for most small burns (less than 5 per cent body surface area).
- Silver sulphadiazine bag for hand burns.
- TETANUS PROPHYLAXIS.
- Routine antibiotics NOT required.
- Review—leave dressing 7–10 days *unless*:
  - —unsure of depth of burn
  - —larger burn
  - —hand burns

First aid

Even minor burns and scalds can be frightening for the patient and relatives. The pain from a relatively superficial burn may be greater than that from a full-thickness burn. First aid consists of removing the burning agent, followed by cold water lavage. In chemical burns copious amounts of water should be used. Do not use too much cold water on very small children, as there is real danger of hypothermia.

The other part of first aid is to give reassurance to the patient and relatives. A calm attitude often relieves most of the anxiety. Some pain relief is required, but simple analgesics, such as paracetamol, are very effective, especially in children.

Assessment

• **History** • **Examination** • **Investigations**

History

Ask the exact nature of the burning agent. The cause of the burn may be easily recognized, but the depth of scald caused by water can range from mild erythema to full-thickness loss. Industrial steam, domestic steam, and water from a boiling kettle or a cup of coffee will all produce different depths of burn for the same time exposure.

Where chemicals are involved the exact nature and concentration of the substance should be sought. Labels on the container are the best guide.

The length of time the skin was in contact with the burning agent is ascertained. The longer the contact time the deeper the burn.

The time elapsed from the burning is of the same importance as for any other wound. If more than six hours have elapsed since the burn then it is more likely that the wound will be infected.

> **The tetanus status must be ascertained. Adequate tetanus prophylaxis is often forgotten in minor burns.**

Allergy is excluded and information is sought on other medications and other medical problems.

Examination

The area of burn is estimated by charting on burns charts or by using the hand of the patient (see pp. 206–207).

The appearance of the burn will give clues to the depth:

- Very superficial burns will exhibit simple erythema
- Superficial burns will have thin-walled blisters
- Deeper burns will blister
- Full-thickness burns will have a leathery, pale appearance

The presence of sensation in the burn area is assessed using a blunt pin, its absence indicating a deep burn.

It can be very difficult to be sure of the depth of a burn, and indeed many deep burns have a mixed depth of injury.

The *general examination* of the patient will depend on the exact circumstances of the burn. A simple scald on the forearm will not normally require a general examination of the whole patient. However, a patient with superficial facial burns from a house fire will require an examination of the upper airways, a general examination, and a chest examination.

Investigations

The majority of minor burns will require no investigations. If smoke inhalation is suspected then blood and radiological investigations may be required (see p. 211). If the burn appears infected then a bacteriological swab may be indicated.

Treatment: burns dressing

- **When to use** • **Wound preparation**
- **Routine dressing** • **Alternative methods**

When to use

This section outlines ONE method of treatment for a *small* (less than 5 per cent), *partial-thickness* burn **not** in a '*special area*' (hand, face, perineum). Local practice will vary, but the treatment given is safe, effective, and cost-efficient.

Most partial-thickness burns can be treated successfully on an out-patient basis. Burns will heal if infection does not supervene. A moist wound environment speeds wound healing. The mainstay of treatment is wound toilet and a 'burns dressing'.

Wound preparation

Simple erythema requires no specific treatment. However, as the blister may take some time to appear, instruct the patient to return if blistering occurs.

The burn blister. There is debate over the best way to deal with a blister. The traditional method was to deroof the blister, but this has been shown to increase bacterial colonization of the burn wound, and makes the pain worse. The blister may be left intact, but if it is large and thin-walled the blister fluid may be aspirated while the blister roof is left intact.

Aseptic technique is used throughout. The burn area is cleaned with sterile saline. If the blister requires aspiration it is pierced using a 19-gauge (white) hypodermic needle, and the blister fluid is removed. Sometimes the blistered skin is almost detached; if this is the case it should be removed. There is no merit in formally removing all the blister skin, as the raw area left is very painful.

Routine dressing

The aim of the dressing is to exclude pathogenic bacteria and to provide a moist wound environment to aid healing. The traditional dressing consists of four layers (Figure 13.1):

(1) a moist non-adherent layer
(2) a dry non-adherent layer
(3) an absorbing layer
(4) a securing layer

(a)

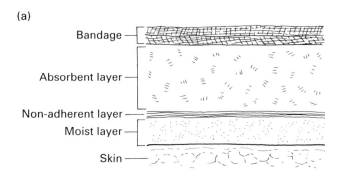

(b)

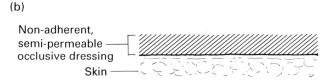

Fig. 13.1 . Burns dressing. (a) Multi-layered method. (b) Single-layered method.

The first layer usually consists of a *paraffin-impregnated gauze* (Paratulle, Bactigras—use in children).

Apply 2–3 layers of the gauze to cover the wound. A single layer will soon dry out and adhere to the wound.

Silver sulphadiazine cream (Flamazine®) is an alternative to the use of gauze.

The second layer is a non-adherent dressing, to separate the wound from the third layer, the absorbent layer. It is important that the exudate from the burn does not reach the outer layers of the dressing. Were this to occur there would be a moist track of a very good culture medium (the burn exudate), which might turn into a gateway for bacterial entry into the wound.

The final layer is to hold the dressing in place. On the limbs this is relatively easy, but for difficult areas, such as the trunk, there is no substitute for the skill and ingenuity of an experienced A&E nurse. Wide-weave cotton bandage (Netelast) is often successful in these areas.

The patient is given tetanus prophylaxis as needed. Analgesia is given (paracetamol is usually effective).

Patients are instructed to keep the dressing dry. If the outer layer becomes wet from the burn exudate then they should return for re-dressing. Otherwise the dressing may be left for 7 to 10 days before the patient is reviewed.

Alternative methods

There are many methods of treating a burn wound, and those given above are simple and well tried. Burns may be treated without any dressing (exposure), but this requires great attention to detail and hygiene.

The variety of types of dressings recommended by manufacturers for dressing of burns is great and growing. There is some evidence that certain types of dressing, such as Opsite and Omniderm, reduce pain more than conventional techniques. There are also claims that healing is faster. The difference would amount to 1–2 days in most burns which are treated in A&E departments.

Undoubtedly, some dressings may have advantages in certain types of burn or patient. Each department will have a policy on the preferred dressing to use.

Other methods of treatment

- **Burns of the hand**
- **Flamazine bag**
- **Burns of the face**
- **Burns of the eyes**

Burns of the hand

These are potentially very serious. Although the area of burn may be small, the skin of the hand is extremely specialized, and full-thickness loss of greater than 1 cm diameter should be referred immediately to the in-patient specialist team. Scars on the hand may give rise to contractures which prevent normal finger function.

For these reasons burns and scalds of the hand require

increased care compared with those of similar depth and size in other parts of the body. However, most burns of the hand can be effectively treated on an out-patient basis as long as these considerations are kept in mind.

It is often difficult to dress hand burns in the normal way. If the hand is immobilized by a bulky dressing for any length of time then there is a likelihood of joint stiffness and prolonged disability. The method of choice in treating large hand burns is the silver sulphadiazine hand bag (Flamazine bag, Figure 13.2).

Flamazine bag

After the usual wound toilet and cleaning the burned areas are covered with silver sulphadiazine cream. The hand is then placed in a polythene bag or glove. The neck of the bag is then taped over gauze at the wrist (Figure 13.2).

The patient is instructed to move the hand actively inside the bag, and also to elevate the hand (proper elevation: see Figure 8.17, p. 163).

There are two problems with this method of treatment. The first is that burn exudate rapidly accumulates in the bag. This makes the bag prone to burst, thus rendering the dressing no longer occlusive. The patient can be given a spare bag and cream in case this should occur. The patient should have the bag replaced every day. If there is excessive exudate then hospital admission may be required.

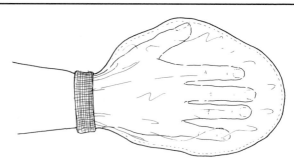

Fig. 13.2 . Flamazine bag.

The other problem is that the normal hand skin soon becomes macerated through being placed in such a moist, enclosed environment. After four or five days the patient will complain about the hand's appearance.

After three to four days it is usually more obvious which areas of the hand will require dressing, and often only one or two fingers will need further occlusion, and a formal 'burns dressing' may be used.

Burns of the face

The common mechanisms of injury causing facial burns/ scalds are the blow-back from a faulty gas appliance or of boiling water from a car radiator.

Isolated serious facial burns are rare. It is vital to recognize the signs which suggest airway involvement (see p. 217).

The eyes should be carefully examined (see below). Any involvement of the cornea or deep burns of the lid margin should be referred for expert opinion.

If the burn is superficial (erythema or very minor blistering) then it may be treated on an out-patient basis. If the burn is more serious than this then admission is advisable.

If the burn is to be treated on an out-patient basis then exposure is the best method.

The wound is cleaned and left open. No other treatment is needed.

Burns of the eyes

The protective reflexes make burns of the eyes fairly rare. The major exception is that of chemical burns, when the reflex actively keeps the burning agent in contact with the eye. Alkali (e.g. cement) burns of the eye are especially serious. If the eye is involved in a burn then accurate examination is essential. The same principles are followed as with other eye wounds.

Burns to the eyes should be immediately triaged into the most urgent category, and receive immediate treatment.

Remove all particulate matter, then irrigate the eye. The instillation of amethocaine may facilitate the procedure. If there has been significant chemical contamination use at least 2 litres of saline, and irrigate to a pH of 7.

The eye is inspected, and any gross abnormality is noted. Pupillary reactions are noted. AN ASSESSMENT OF VISUAL ACUITY MUST BE MADE. This part of the examination is often neglected, but is one of the most sensitive indicators of serious damage.

Assess the clarity of the cornea; any haziness indicates a severe burn. Look for loss of any blood vessels over the conjunctiva, especially around the limbus.

The cornea is then stained with fluorescein and examined with cobalt-blue light to show any areas of epithelial loss.

If there is a burn then some chloramphenicol ointment is applied, a mydriatic (cyclopentolate) is instilled, and the eye is covered. The patient is then referred immediately to the ophthalmologists. All significant alkali burns must be referred immediately, since the damage caused by such agents may mean total loss of sight.

Deep burns of the lid margins may lead to scarring, resulting in entropion or ectropion.

Index